S0-ACO-312

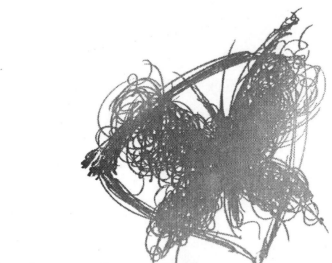

Touched by Grace

Ruth Penner

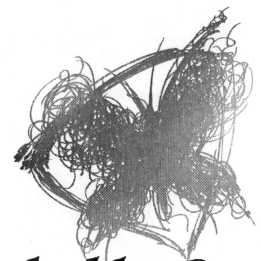

Touched by Grace
From Secrecy
to New Life

Ann Showalter
Foreword by John Weborg

DreamSeeker Books
TELFORD, PENNSYLVANIA

an imprint of
Cascadia Publishing House

Copublished with
Herald Press
Scottdale, Pennsylvania

Cascadia Publishing House orders, information, reprint permissions:
contact@CascadiaPublishingHouse.com
1-215-723-9125
126 Klingerman Road, Telford PA 18969
www.CascadiaPublishingHouse.com

Touched By Grace
Copyright © 2006 by Cascadia Publishing House.
Telford, PA 18969
All rights reserved
DreamSeeker Books is an imprint of Cascadia Publishing House.
Copublished with Herald Press, Scottdale, PA
Library of Congress Catalog Number: 2005021753
ISBN: 1-931038-33-3
Book design by Cascadia Publishing House
Cover design by Gwen M. Stamm

The paper used in this publication is recycled and meets the
minimum requirements of American National Standard for Information Sciences—
Permanence of Paper for Printed Library Materials, ANSI Z39.48-1984.1984

All Bible quotations are used by permission, all rights reserved and unless
otherwise noted are from *The New Revised Standard Version of the Bible*, copyright 1989, by the Division of Christian Education of the National Council
of the Churches of Christ in the USA.

Library of Congress Cataloguing-in-Publication Data
Showalter, Ann.
Touched by grace : from secrecy to new life / Ann Showalter ; foreword by John
Weborg.
    p. cm.
ISBN-13: 978-1-931038-33-1 (trade pbk. : alk. paper)
ISBN-10: 1-931038-33-3 (trade pbk. : alk. paper)
1. Showalter, Ray E., 1929- 2. AIDS (Disease)--Patients--Biography. I. Title.
RC607.A26S494 2006
362.196'9792'0092--dc22

                                                    2005021753

12 11 10 09 08 07 06   10 9 8 7 6 5 4 3 2

*To the memory
of my husband Ray
and to our four children*

Contents

PART THREE

PART FOUR

Foreword

Ann Showalter has written a book about "discoveries become episodes of biography, unpredictable as the new world the discoverers opened to us" (Daniel Boorstin, *The Discoverers: A History of Man's Search to Know His World and Himself,* Random House, 1983, p. xv). "The discovery unpredictable" was that her husband was dying of AIDS, that he had wrestled with the sexual orientation of his person since youth, that he had actively participated in such relationships while married, and that his activity was unknown to Ann until weeks before her husband died. Retrospectively she could see the pattern in their marriage of a reluctant intimacy, of an avoidance latent in overwork and a diminishing spontaneity. These discoveries became episodes of biography (her husband) and of an autobiography (herself).

Ann's book is neither journal nor diary, although it contains elements of both, especially journal entries. Her work is candid, capable of truthful, direct engagement with the discovered episodes of a life together that remained largely unnamed until shortly before her husband's death. The telling of his story is neither voyeuristic nor exploitative, and always with the consent of the people involved: their children and the time the family assembled to hear a husband and father reveal history;

the friends and community with which Ann's husband had shared much of his life; the extended family; finally, the larger communities in which the Showalters had been participants.

The direct yet thorough manner in which Ann relates these encounters finds delicate description in the poignant phrasing of Emmanuel Levinas:

> Alliterate (the "otherwise" of another) becomes proximity. Not distance, the shortest through space, but initial directness, which extends as unimpeachable approach in the call of the face of the other, in which there appears, as an order, an inscription, a prescription, an awakening (as if it were a "me"), responsibility—mine, for another human being. The face of the other, in its defenseless nakedness—is it not already (despite the countenance this baseness may put on) an asking. (Emmanuel Levinas, *In the Time of the Nations*, trans. Michael B. Smith, University of Indiana Press, 1994, p. 110; cf. p. 26)

Ann knows the power of the phrase "proximity to otherness"—husband, family of origin, nuclear family, extended family, church families—churches of origin and current participation. Each of the communities and special persons within them needed to be faced and told the news of her husband's impending death and its precipitating causes. Levinas again: "The face of the other, in its defenseless nakedness—is it not already . . . an asking?" Repeated settings and narrative, each with a nuanced change in the telling, allowed the story to grow into a more complete form. As Levinas says, the evocative phenomenon is owed to "the call of the face of the other," "in its defenseless nakedness" yet with vulnerability receptive to a directness of speech accompanied by devotion interchanged between speaker and listener.

As for Ann, discoveries continued to become episodes of biography and autobiography. Like letting gifts for ministry mature by means of a theological education. Like letting Clinical Pastoral Education serve as both critical and caring experiences. Like permitting herself to tell her story in grief recovery groups. Like letting herself be introduced to the world of gay men and lesbian women, to hear stories of deep hurt, of alienation from families and religious communities—to experience the defenseless nakedness of the face.

Ann looked long and intensely into these faces and felt a claim from them and a call from God. She took up a ministry in the AIDS Pastoral Care Network and found herself in the Lord's vineyard of AIDS education and a ministry to the terminally ill and the bereaved. The story of Abraham, leaving everything familiar and facing everything unfamiliar, became her companion in her effort to be at home in a country not of her choosing but of her calling. She embraced it the same way Abraham did, by faith.

Along the way, Ann lets the reader overhear her own conversations and prayers about matters that are complicated, vexed, painful, and controversial. She invites our company, not necessarily our consent. It's a very good company to be in because when any reader comes face to face with "discoveries become episodes of biography" Ann's itinerary will help in spotting the landmarks.

— *John Weborg*
Twenty-Fourth Week of Pentecost

Preface

The book you hold in your hand is a personal story of love, commitment to God and the church, and serving others. It is a story of suffering, betrayal, and a hidden life. It is a story of truth-telling, compassion, redemption, reconciliation, healing, and finally my husband's death from AIDS.

We were parents of four adult children. The book leaves unanswered the questions many people have regarding the long-term response of our children to the discovery of their father's sexual orientation and hidden life. Leaving such questions unanswered is intentional because that is not my story to tell but theirs.

I hope as you read the book you will discover that its *central* theme is not the details of my husband's death or of my complicated grief or my work with people directly affected by AIDS— but the *grace of God* that creates newness amid tragedy and death.

—*Ann Showalter*
Newton, Kansas

Acknowledgments

Within the first year after the death of my husband, friends began urging me to write the story of his illness and death. It was too early. I knew I had to heal first, but I didn't know it would be fifteen years before I would be ready to undertake the project.

Even then, I'm not sure this book ever would have been started without the encouragement of my longtime friend Norma Sutton. "You come to my house and we will write," she invited. She furnished her family room with a bed and a computer and all I needed to be comfortable. For six weeks she cooked my food, washed my clothes, and was available to critique and encourage me. Her gifts to me were beyond price.

After a three-year interruption, I continued the writing in the company of the sisters at Heartland Center for Spirituality in Great Bend, Kansas. Their hospitality, interest, and encouragement created an atmosphere in which writing became a pleasure. Sister Louise Hageman, my spiritual director at Heartland, believed in me and in the importance of my writing. To her I offer my heartfelt thanks.

Walter Friesen, a psychologist, pastor, and friend, gave hours and hours to reading, correcting, and organizing the manuscript. Reflecting together on various aspects of the writing stimulated my thinking and often gave me the courage to continue writing when I felt like the manuscript might never be completed.

Additional credit and thanks go to Father Jim Corrigan, Patrick Hanson, Cheryl Young, Mark Siemens, and Anna Juhnke, who read parts or all of the manuscript and offered suggestions that have made this a far better book than it could have become without their help and encouragement.

Gordon Houser deserves credit and my thanks for the initial editing of the manuscript so that it was presentable for sample chapters to go to the publisher and later the full manuscript to Mark Siemens, who did the final editing before his untimely death of a stroke. Mark encouraged me from his first reading of the partly completed manuscript. His words gave me the necessary courage and patience to keep trying to find a publisher when I thought it might never happen. I'm especially grateful for Mark's persistence in pushing for clarity of thought, his gracious manner in the way that was done, and his ability to make the editorial task a genuinely collaborative effort.

The loving support of my children through these many years alone has meant more to me than they will ever know.

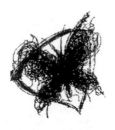

Part One

Do not fear, for I have redeemed you;
I have called you by name, you are mine.
When you pass through the waters, I will be with you;
and through the rivers, they shall not overwhelm you;
when you walk through fire you shall not be burned,
and the flame shall not consume you.
For I am the LORD your God,
the Holy One of Israel, your Savior.
—Isaiah 43:1b–3a

1

June 1984

Forebodings

June 1, 1984, is fixed in my mind forever. I was driving from Park Ridge, Illinois, to my home in Oak Park, a Chicago suburb, and reviewing the events of the day. Without warning a message of startling clarity burst into awareness. *Ann, you have to confront what is going on with Ray.* The words were as clear as if spoken audibly though, of course, they weren't. The message arrived full-blown, not from conscious thought. Intuitively I recognized it as from the Spirit, whose quiet voice I had learned to recognize and trust after many years of seeking God or, more accurately, responding to God seeking me.

Since late the previous fall, I had been aware of changes in Ray, my husband. At first the changes were subtle. He slept more on weekends, lost a few pounds, and often suggested we share a meal when we ate out. Ray had always worked long hours and caught up on sleep on weekends whenever possible. And he had been careful about his weight for years. These changes were a matter of degree. As the winter progressed, it became clear he was not feeling well. He frequently took medication. Several times I inquired about his health only to be rebuffed soundly. "You really don't need to worry about me. I can take care of myself. After all, I am a nurse." My stress increased as his silence and my concern for his health became more acute.

While preparing dinner, I reflected on the message that jolted me earlier. I decided to wait until after dinner when there was plenty of time to talk in a relaxed atmosphere before approaching Ray. He was stretched out on the living room floor watching TV after I had finished cleaning up the kitchen. The time had come.

"Ray," I said, "I know something has been going on with you. I don't know what it is, but I have to know." I was not used to making such forceful and direct requests of my husband. I had grown up in a home in which my father issued the ultimatums. However, the clarity and force of that earlier message gave me the permission and confidence to request and expect an answer from him.

"Get down here with me, and I'll tell you," Ray said. I lay beside him on the floor. "Since early January, I have been under my doctor's care. My blood platelet count is dangerously low, and I am scheduled for a bone marrow biopsy on Monday."

"What in the world are they looking for, leukemia?"

"I don't know, I guess so."

"I want to go with you on Monday."

"No! There's no reason for you to go. I'm going straight from work. There's no reason for you to go along."

"But there is. I'm your wife."

"No! You aren't going."

I knew further argument was useless.

That Friday evening, June 1, 1984, my world shattered, turned upside down. You could also say my world was beginning to turn right side up.

Even though I capitulated to his determination to go alone for the biopsy, my firm request was like a practice run in assertiveness. I did not know it was only the first of many tough requests I would make of Ray in the weeks ahead.

On June 3, I wrote in my journal:

I feel less need to determine how Ray will deal with this crisis. Much as I wanted to go to the doctor with him, I realize I must give him the space he wants. Dealing with something as personal as a catastrophic illness deserves the greatest respect for the wishes and needs of the person. It is not a time to capitalize on my own needs. I feel a great tenderness—a desire to take care of him, yet knowing that is my need, not his. We have some tender, touching moments. Not many words, but a touch of the hands and a sense of being close.

On Monday Ray went to the doctor while I waited at home. When he returned, he was carrying a new suit he had picked up after having it altered. "I'll probably never wear this except in my coffin," he said morbidly. I thought he was being overly dramatic.

He was to go back to the doctor for the biopsy report on Thursday afternoon. He had become increasingly worried about his health, examining his legs before dressing each morning and checking them again in the evening. One of his ankles was swollen, and he appeared to have less energy.

Usually we drove to work together. He was at the wheel until we arrived at his office, then I drove back across the city to my office. That week, however, he asked me to do all the driving. Since I worked only Monday, Wednesday, and Friday, he rode the El on Tuesday and drove on Thursday. We fretted in silence, talking little as we waited for Thursday.

Thursday morning, before Ray left for work, I pled to go with him to the doctor's office. It was useless. He was adamant. No way would he consent to my going along. His appointment was at five. He went directly from work as planned. Seven o'-clock came and went, and he had not returned. I became more and more anxious as time passed. When he still was not home at eight, I called Bob, a chaplain friend, who lived nearby.

Ray returned shortly after Bob arrived. The biopsy report contained good and bad news. The bone marrow was producing healthy blood platelets and red cells as it does normally. However, the platelets were being destroyed in the blood stream. The doctor ordered Ray to report for admission to Illinois Masonic Hospital on Sunday afternoon, June 10, for comprehensive medical examinations. All signs pointed to something serious, but I had no idea what. Ray said that if the illness proved to be irreversible, he would not seek unusual measures to stay alive. I felt relieved. In my work as a hospital chaplain, I had seen the horrible consequences of heroics. Yet my anxiety escalated when he said "irreversible illness."

Bob read Scripture and prayed with us before leaving. I felt reassured that whatever lay ahead, God would walk beside us. God would not leave us alone.

Ray worked on Friday and rested most of Saturday. In the evening he insisted I drive him to his office so he could work several hours before going to the hospital the next day. He was not one to leave loose ends for someone else to tie up. He worked only in spurts and rested between. He labored for every breath.

As usual we attended Sunday morning worship with the Oak Park Mennonite Church. The congregation was small, and it was customary to share "joys and concerns" with the group during worship. Ray told the group he was going into the hospital that afternoon for a thorough medical examination, and the group prayed for us.

I was somber as we went home for lunch. Without our choice we were starting a new and frightening journey, and I was anxious, not knowing what the future held. I could not imagine how it would transform my life.

Admission to the hospital was completed quickly. Almost before Ray could get into bed a medical resident arrived to take a medical history and perform the initial physical examination. He asked me to leave the room. I complied but was seething inside, much as I had when I felt overpowered by authority as a child. Why all the secrecy? Does the doctor assume I have never seen my husband's body in more than thirty-one years of marriage? I went home and waited.

The tests continued through the week. I visited briefly each day. On Thursday afternoon he was to undergo a bronchoscopy, an uncomfortable, invasive procedure that is performed in surgery under anesthetic.

A note in my journal reflects my confusion:

My feelings about Ray's illness are so mixed. Sometimes I'm angry for he drives himself so hard. He lives with too much stress, yet I am helpless to change any of that. I'm sad, incredibly sad, that we have not been best friends as well as husband and wife. I wonder how long it will be until we are given a diagnosis? How long will his recovery be? What if it is something that can't be treated?

During a visit with my therapist that week, I told him Ray was in the hospital.

"I'm afraid he will work himself to death some day," I said.

"Let's suppose he does," the therapist responded. "Imagine for a few minutes that he dies. What will you do? Whom do you want at the bedside? What kind of a service will you plan? I want you to think through and talk through the whole process."

I was horrified. "I can't do that!"

"Yes, you can. Do it!" He was not about to let me off the hook. I collected my thoughts for few minutes, then described in detail what I would do.

2

Speaking the Truth

When I visited Ray on Saturday afternoon, he asked me to call our pastor, Ardean, to come for a visit. Ardean promised to arrive around three. As three approached, I prepared to leave, assuming the pastor's visit was to be as private as the visits of the medical residents had been, but Ray asked me to stay. I was so glad.

Pastor Ardean arrived with Norma, his wife. She rarely made hospital visits with Ardean but decided at the last minute to come. The four of us were good friends. "Raise the head of the bed, please," Ray said. I did. It was easier for him to see Ardean and Norma. He quickly got to the business at hand.

"I have something to tell you that scares me a lot," he said, "because it will hurt you, especially Ann. I have AIDS."

I have AIDS. Those three short words are seared indelibly into my heart and mind. I dropped my head to rest on the edge of his bed. It took about fifteen seconds for my brain to compute two things: Ray had been sexually active outside our marriage, and he was going to die.

"You don't have to stay with me if you don't want to," he said. "I can get someone else to take care of me."

"Why would I leave you now?" Although the words came quickly I knew I meant them.

Ardean and Norma were at the bedside with me, but neither said a word. Ray spoke without further interruption, unhurried, deliberately, as if wanting to get into the open something that had been hidden a long time.

"I have lived as a gay man in recent years," he said.

"Finally, the pieces of the puzzle fit together," I said. Most of what followed these initial statements I do not recall. At one point I said, "All I know is that from now on, things will have to be put on the table in a different way than they have been."

When Ray had finished his story, Ardean stepped to the bedside, took both of Ray's hands into his own, looked him straight in the eyes and said, "I love you, brother." What a moment! I can imagine no words more appropriate or more healing, no response more Christlike.

I cried quietly after Ray's opening words. Following Ardean's response, my grief overwhelmed me. I asked Ardean to leave the room with me. Norma stayed with Ray. Ardean found a small storage room filled with chairs. We sat in privacy and he held me while I wept my heart out. As my sobbing subsided, grief was replaced by rage, waves of rage like I had never known.

"I have to leave the hospital," I said. "I can't stay here any longer."

We went back into Ray's room, and I said good-bye to him. Norma came with me and Ardean stayed with Ray. Ardean told me much later that he and Ray had quite a prayer meeting after Norma and I had left.

My thoughts raced wildly as Norma and I walked across the parking lot to my car. This is like a soap opera, I thought. Yet I knew it was no soap opera; it was my life, as real as anything could possibly be, hard as that was for me to believe. I realized I had already lived through the pain of the years Ray had been living a double life; there was no need to spend energy reliving that pain. Too much of immediate importance captured my attention to dwell on the past. I also thought, *Ann, you are so fortunate to be living in Chicago instead of a small rural town.* I remembered how vigorously I had resisted moving to Chicago in 1980.

Somewhere in the mix of things I became aware of God's providential care. The crisis I faced could not have come at a more appropriate time in terms of my professional and ministerial preparation. Ray had stood at my side two weeks earlier as I took my ordination vows. The week Ray was hospitalized I had signed a one-year contract with Associated Mennonite Biblical Seminaries (now Seminary) in Elkhart, Indiana, with the option of staying longer if I wished to. Another thought flashed across my mental screen: We could not be in a better place in terms of the support of a faith community as well as professional support. I was grateful.

Norma slipped into the driver's seat of my car as I closed the door on the passenger side. I pounded my fist on the dashboard. "Finally, I know I have not been crazy all these years." It was a moment of great lucidity, a self-defining moment. I felt a physical sensation through the center of my body as if someone had slipped a strong, straight brace along my spine that fit perfectly. Suddenly I knew who I was in a way I had never known before. The awareness stayed with me throughout that eventful summer, and the memory of that moment continues to sustain me.

In amazement I wondered, *How is it possible that a woman who is part of a faith tradition that condemns homosexuality as sin finds herself in the middle of Chicago with a gay husband who is dying of AIDS?* It is a long story.

Night is an apt metaphor for the darkness I felt long before the sun disappeared beyond the western horizon. Norma went with me to our home in Oak Park for the night. She screened telephone calls and listened to me hour after hour. She did not pry in any way but listened with care and understanding. She accepted without criticism my outbursts of anger as well as my sadness as I grappled with the tragedy of the diagnosis. Before going to bed, she invited me to call her if I woke during the night and wanted to talk. The night that followed sunset seemed endless.

I took her at her word and woke her in the early morning hours, the hours that seem longest when one is in crisis. As I talked, I realized that Ray had also suffered during our marriage, not only when my critical attitudes and anger surfaced but from his own conflicts related to his sexual orientation.

When morning came, I called a Catholic priest friend to tell him about Ray's diagnosis. Father Jim Corrigan was one of my supervisors during my residency in Clinical Pastoral Education (CPE) following my graduation from seminary.

I had entered CPE with three other students at Rush-Presbyterian—St. Luke's Medical Center in Chicago on September 1, 1982. Early in the program each of us shared our spiritual journey with the group. Jim supervised the group. Since there were only five of us, we spoke candidly. Each of us took one class period to tell our story. Jim took his turn last. He sat cross-legged in his chair. Pushing up his sleeves and crossing his arms over his chest, he said, "I am a gay man!" His words hit me like a fist to the chest, taking my breath away. The next instant I realized Jim was a person with whom I could share my growing suspicion that Ray was gay, without the fear he would be judged harshly. At the close of his story, Jim assured us he would not continue referring to his being gay. Instead, he invited us to initiate conversation with him if at any time we had questions.

Jim was also my individual supervisor. Several weeks went by before I had the courage to say, "Jim, sometime I want to talk with you about what you told us in your spiritual journey." I could not bring myself to say "gay" or "homosexual." He said, "Whenever you are ready." It was enough. Several weeks later in conference, I said, "Jim, I think my husband is gay." By the time I choked the words from my mouth, I was sobbing.

Jim sat quietly, allowing me plenty of time to cry. Then he gently touched my foot with his and said, "Ann, if that's the case, it has nothing to do with you. That was there long before Ray knew you." His words, though few, lifted an enormous burden from me. For years I had felt it was my fault Ray had little interest in me as a woman. Jim understood the feelings of rejection and isolation that come when our sexual identity is not accepted or validated. As our conversation ended, he offered to be available if I ever needed pastoral care related to homosexuality.

In the months that followed, I thought often of Jim's words and the burden they had lifted. I clung to them, drawing from them every bit of relief and self-acceptance I could. I pondered the power of words: some give comfort and hope, others pierce the heart like a sword. But even those can become a source of hope when they speak the truth. Ray's words—"I have AIDS"—hit me like heavy blows, but the truth they spoke soon became a breath of fresh air. In the weeks that followed, Ray's words liberated both of us from old bonds of deception and secrecy. Jim's words freed me from a great weight of inadequacy and shame. Ardean's words—"I love you, brother"—spoke of genuine acceptance and became redemptive words for Ray.

When I called Jim that Sunday morning to tell him about Ray, he cautioned me to choose carefully whom to share Ray's diagnosis with. "Once you tell someone, you can never take it back," he warned.

In his work as a hospital chaplain, Jim saw young men suffering the ravages of AIDS. He was well aware of the pervasive fear that affected almost everyone who came in contact with or heard of a person with AIDS. What has now become a worldwide scourge was a recent phenomenon in the Midwest at the time Ray was stricken. The virus now referred to as the Human Immunodeficiency Virus (HIV) had not yet been identified with certainty in June 1984.

It was not difficult to take Jim's advice. I felt so utterly shattered that I needed time to live with the truth myself before sharing it beyond a few close friends. Although I appreciated and trusted the people in our church, I was not prepared to attend worship there and reveal Ray's diagnosis. Instead Norma and I attended Roman Catholic Mass in the chapel at Rush-Presbyterian—St. Luke's Medical Center, where I had worked as a chaplain the previous year. We ate lunch in the atrium lunchroom at the hospital before Norma returned to her home and I went to Illinois Masonic Hospital to visit Ray.

3
_____

Starting a
New Life Together

My earlier conversations with Norma had prepared me to visit Ray with compassion in my heart. Though I felt betrayed and angry, I still loved Ray. I wanted to assure him of my love and let him know I wanted him to come home if he got well enough. Later I recorded in my journal what I told him that afternoon.

> Ray, let me say this much. I do not see you as a bad person. You have contributed much to my life, and there is nothing that happens to us that God cannot use for good. That doesn't mean I'm not hurt and angry and enormously sad. It does mean I love you and accept you as a very precious human being. What has happened cannot negate our more than thirty-one years of marriage or the fact that we have raised a family of four children. I too have often failed to live up to the commitments we made to each other and surely have hurt you in many ways.

Although Ray did not respond with words, he seemed happy to see me, and I felt his appreciation.

Naturally, I wondered if I had been exposed to the virus. Apart from reading a few newspaper articles about a new disease primarily affecting gay men, my knowledge of AIDS was nil.

Ray's primary physician, Dr. David Moore, stopped in to see him while I was at the bedside. I had not met him before. His manner was unhurried as he examined Ray then stayed to visit. It was reassuring to observe his attention not only to Ray's physical well-being but to his emotional state as well.

Later I looked for Dr. Moore as I had a number of questions. I soon found him in a conference room, and he immediately invited me to take a chair across the table from him. I asked if I was in danger while visiting Ray. (There was a notice outside Ray's room that specified wearing a mask and gown before entering.) I was relieved to learn the mask and gown were unnecessary except when exposure to blood or other body fluids was likely. Dr. Moore confirmed that I could have been exposed to the virus before Ray's admission but suggested there was only a slim chance of my developing AIDS, since most people who had contracted AIDS in our country at the time had a history of other sexually transmitted diseases. (We now know this is not always true.) I also found some consolation when he told me very few women had been diagnosed. I was less comforted to hear that the medical community did not know the length of the incubation period or the duration of the infectious stage of the virus. My fear of infection was most alleviated because our intimate contact had been quite limited for many months. How ironic that our limited and less-than-satisfying sex may well have saved my life.

In June 1984 no test was available to determine whether or not I had been infected with the virus. Furthermore, there were no effective drugs available to slow or halt the replication of the virus. Drugs could temporarily clear up some of the diseases that develop when the immune system is compromised, but they had no effect against the virus. I asked myself how I would live my life differently if I knew I was infected and discovered there was nothing I would change except perhaps move closer to our children. Even that seemed unlikely and impractical, since they were scattered from south-central Kansas to Texas and Mississippi. Unlikely though it may sound even to me, I never lost any sleep because of fear of infection. Three years later when a test was available, my doctor asked me to take it. Since I was scheduled for minor surgery that could possibly pose a threat to someone else, I agreed. The result was negative, no evidence of the virus.

When and how should we tell our children the diagnosis? Ray had called each of them to tell them he was being admitted to the hospital for diagnostic work. It was important to me that Ray tell them, but I wondered if I should wait until he improved. Dr. Moore agreed that Ray should be the person to tell the children. He did not think it wise to wait, since AIDS can be unpredictable. I left feeling heard, supported, and more informed.

Soon after I returned to Ray's room, a man entered with a vase of elegant, white orchids. Ray introduced us. I recognized Bill's name as the person Ray had dinner with on Tuesday evenings when I worked late, but our paths had never crossed. Meeting Bill face-to-face at Ray's bedside was uncomfortable. I imagined all kinds of painful scenarios but could not judge whether they were realistic. I needed to go home.

Later I told Ray he was welcome to have his gay friends visit him when I was not there—he needed all the support he could get—but they could not be present when I was visiting. He promised it would not happen again and it didn't.

At home I prayed:

> God, I don't know where to go from here. What will happen to Ray? He has been my husband for thirty-one and a half years. How can all those years be treated as nothing? They can't. He's been good to me in many ways. He's even loved me as much as he was capable of loving any woman. He has suffered much and is suffering now. Please be with him to make this a positive experience of healing for him. Let him know he is loved.

Sin runs so deep and the costs are so high. Is Ray going to live? Will he continue his homosexual involvement? God, I don't know the answer to any of these questions. God, will I be able to live the rest of my life without sex? Can Ray and I reconcile? How do we begin?

Ray usually had shown his love with thoughtful, generous gifts. He always made sure I had enough money in my purse for household needs. We enjoyed working together when we were entertaining guests. I counted on him to set a beautiful table while I gave my attention to preparing the food. He taught me to appreciate order and beauty, good music and art, the theater and ballet. He had enriched my life in many ways.

It was the limited emotional support, the almost total absence of sharing thoughts and feelings, and the dearth of affection that became so painful. Most of the time I did not feel my femininity was valued or of interest to him. Intimacy seemed like more of an obligation than a passionate desire for a close physical relationship.

As I reflected on our relationship, I felt certain he must have carried a heavy load through the years, knowing he was gay while also knowing the condemnation that would come his way if people at work and in the church ever discovered his secret. How could I reestablish trust, and how could I let go of my anger so we could relate respectfully?

I called each of our children that evening to let them know their father was very ill, but I chose not to tell them the diagnosis. I said, "We need to spend time together as a family. I want all of you here next weekend." I will never know how difficult that week was for them, waiting and waiting without knowing what they would face when they arrived in Chicago.

The big item on the next day's agenda was to tell Ray I expected him to tell the children his diagnosis. I began, "You said the other day that no one else needs to know about the diagnosis, that it's no one else's business. It *is* someone else's business. Our children need to know, and they need to know it from you."

"They can't afford to come to Chicago."

"Look, they are all adults. They will find the money somewhere. I have already called them. They are all coming next weekend." I could see my words dealt him a blow. Later in the day he called me at home and offered to write a letter he wanted me to read to them over the telephone.

"No. We need to be together," I insisted. "They are coming next weekend."

I, too, dreaded the moment of truth when Ray would tell them. I had no idea how to plan for the occasion. Would he want them all together or would he rather tell them individually? Would he want me present or not? Should the pastor be on standby? How would the kids react? In midweek over lunch with Jim Corrigan, I told him about my concerns. "Why don't you ask Ray what he wants?" It made perfect sense once he said it, but I would not have thought of it.

My sister, Elizabeth, also lived in Chicago. She had visited Ray before coming to our home in Oak Park on Monday evening. "Ray still doesn't know if you *really* want him to come home if he gets well enough to," she said.

"But I've told him several times I love him and want him to come home."

Apparently he was not convinced.

Early the next morning I went to the hospital, arriving before his breakfast time. The window shades were still drawn, and he had withdrawn into himself. Once more I said, "Ray I still love you and I do want you to come home when you are able. Whether or not you continue to live as a gay man and whether or not we can live together are two separate questions."

Immediately, I was aware I had overstated my feelings. I had no idea what it would be like to live with him and have him continue his sexual relationships with men. The point I wanted to make was that he was welcome to come home whenever that became medically feasible.

With great effort, he said, "Thank you, thank you."

It is impossible to imagine the extreme fatigue and weakness of a person with Pneumocystis carinii pneumonia—one of the infections that signals full-blown AIDS—until you see it firsthand. Bathing, washing hair, brushing teeth, and getting into fresh pajamas required most of a forenoon.

Once Ray had completed his morning care and was resting in a clean bed, I took a good look at the flowers in his room. A large credenza was loaded with flowers from professional colleagues and friends. It was time to discard the flowers that were wilted and create fresh, new arrangements with those that remained. Ray coached me from his bed. "Give the lily on the left a little tug. Put the red rose next to the white carnation. No, actually that will look better in the bouquet at the far end." Ray always had a flair for flower arranging that I could not begin to match. We created new beauty to enjoy.

With each flower I threw away, I was throwing away betrayal, deception, fear, blame, resentment, and self-righteousness: things that had spoiled the dreams we had when we were first married. But we had already begun creating something new and beautiful because we were talking more honestly and openly. To heal all the hurt would take years to complete.

When lunch was over we took naps. I settled into a comfortable chair at the bedside and fell asleep in minutes. Opening my eyes a half-hour later, I sensed the quietness in the room. The peacefulness was almost palpable, such a contrast to the way I often had experienced silences between us in the past. I scarcely moved a muscle, not knowing whether Ray was awake. Then he spoke softly, "It is so peaceful in here." Our spirits were in tune with each other in a remarkable way, something we had experienced far too rarely. What a paradox that we found such peace when we were facing a shortened future together!

Now that Ray's monster was out of the closet and we were speaking the truth to each other, his violation of our marriage vows moved down the scale of what was important to me. The truth, though shocking and infuriating, had set me free.

I said, "Ray I still love you and want to be with you, but I also feel sad, betrayed, angry.

Ray said, "I can understand that." That Ray recognized the validity of my feelings was healing for me. I discovered that when I expressed my painful feelings honestly, my heart had room for love. Our day together was like a rare jewel I will cherish as long as I live.

Evening came and I prepared to leave for home. I was exhausted after nearly twelve hours in the hospital. As I said good night, Ray said, "One of these times we need to talk about the disposal of the body." Five days after diagnosis and Ray suggests a conversation about "disposal of the body." Nothing in our past relationship had prepared me for such directness from Ray.

"Must we do that now or can it wait until later?"

"It can wait until later," he said, but kept talking. I sensed that it could not wait until later. The hour with my therapist the week before flashed into my mind. I sat on the bed and faced him. I said, "This is what I've been thinking. . . ." I described in detail what I had told the therapist. Ray suggested several minor changes. We were surprised by the similarity of our thoughts and plans.

I was in a state of euphoria as I left him for the night. I was aware of the incongruity, the radical contradiction of my joy after planning Ray's funeral. I was also aware that just beneath the surface was an ocean of grief, for all the wasted years we had lived hidden from each other, afraid to share our truth, living as strangers under the same roof. For years I had wondered how we would cope if either of us were facing a terminal illness. Would we remain in hiding? I was unable to imagine how I could survive such a time if there were no more openness than we experienced in our daily life together. Is it any wonder I was euphoric?

4

Speaking the Truth
to the Families

I met three of our four children at O'Hare International Airport on Friday evening. Our third daughter, Carmen, was scheduled to arrive at ten on Saturday morning.

Ray said he wanted us to come directly to the hospital from the airport on Friday evening. He also said he wanted me to be with him when he told the children the truth. Once the preliminary greetings were over, I sat on the bed next to Ray on the side nearest the wall. Tom and Karen stood on the opposite side of the bed, and Krista, who had followed her father into the nursing profession, positioned herself at the foot.

Ray clung to my hand. "I have AIDS," he said. Before he had time to say more, Tom and Karen stepped closer to him and said, almost in unison: "It doesn't matter, you are still our dad." Krista was silent. By the time Ray completed his story, I could feel her anger. We did not linger long. Ray looked exhausted, and the rest of us needed time to mull over what he had told us.

A similar scene developed on Saturday morning when Carmen arrived. Upon hearing the diagnosis, she moved close to Ray, took both his hands into hers, and crossed them over his heart. "You didn't throw me out when I disappointed you, and I'm not going to throw you out." Ray was almost overcome with emotion by her response.

Although it was not an easy weekend for any of us, being together as a family was of crucial importance. We made several visits to the hospital during the weekend. On Saturday afternoon we received permission for Ray to go to the hospital lobby to see and hold our six-month-old grandson. As the children said their good-byes before leaving for their respective homes, they knew it was their final farewell to their father, except for Karen. She asked that I call her in time for her to return to be with Ray once more before he died. It was impossible to know when that would be.

Tom and Carmen had to leave early to get back to work, while Krista and Karen were able to stay a few days with me to engage the services of a funeral director. We chose a casket and determined the appropriate procedures to follow at the time of death. We also arranged for the body to be transported to Kansas by air. A phone call to the mortuary was all that was needed when death came later. I was so grateful for the loving support and assistance of our children.

Ray and I agreed that his body would be taken to Kansas for burial and a memorial service. He wanted to be buried where his parents, grandparents, and a host of other relatives were buried. Together we planned a memorial service to be celebrated in Oak Park after I returned from Kansas.

Another matter of grave concern to me was the cost of medical care. How would I be able to pay the hospital bill with the relatively small amount of hospitalization insurance we carried? I was not willing to find myself alone without financial resources at the end of Ray's life. We had no large assets—only a small "nest egg." The children had been away from home for just a few years, and we were entering what would have been our best earning years. I was scared. My anger and fear motivated me to explore possibilities for protecting the assets if medical costs exceeded the $150,000 cap of our insurance.

Before she left for her home, Krista and I sought legal advice on how our assets could be protected. We discovered that nothing could be done short of a divorce. The attorney suggested that such proceedings, if pursued, should begin well before the insurance policy was exhausted. Furthermore, he felt sure that, under the circumstances, any judge would rule in my favor regarding division of assets. He also said I could remain as closely involved with Ray's care as I wished.

I did not know how I could consider divorce. I had given my heart to Ray many years earlier and had never taken it back although there were times when I was tempted to. I was totally committed to staying close to him until the end. Krista and I discussed the option of divorce. Later I told Ray about my fears and reported what the attorney told us. I assured him I would stay with him to the end even if divorce proved to be the only way to protect what we had earned together through years of hard work. We agreed that when the hospital costs reached $50,000, I would file for divorce. It was a mutual decision of love, yet it felt like a horrible, almost unthinkable option.

Meanwhile, Ray's physical condition changed rapidly, fluctuating dramatically. It was like riding a roller coaster. He could appear to be doing reasonably well one day and the next he could be frighteningly close to death. His physicians ordered what seemed like endless rounds of tests to stay abreast of infections that could quickly become life-threatening. Ray's body, with his poorly functioning immune system, was like a house without roof or window panes, open to every kind of storm, theft, and vandalism. Critical protection was gone. The virus had destroyed his defense against an array of infections the body normally resists.

After Ray realized that neither the children nor I were going to turn our backs on him, his demeanor changed markedly. He was open in ways I had never seen before. He expressed his love for me more readily and more frequently than at any time I could remember. It was equally obvious that he was able to receive my affection in a new and wonderful way. The old barrier so often felt between us was gone. His mask was off; we could be real. The change made me more fully aware of just how deeply his secret had affected our lives. It seemed like it had created crippling divisions within Ray and painful distance between us.

Within days after the children's visit, Ray said, "What do you think about inviting Bob and Doris (a brother and sister-in-law) to come for a weekend?"

"I don't understand, why do you want them to come?"

"I want to talk with Bob about some business matters."

"That's up to you, it's fine with me if you want them to come."

Was this really happening? Was I hearing right? What I heard was almost impossible to believe. This man, my husband, who all his life had vigorously protected his privacy, now considered allowing members of his family into his life. He knew that if they came he would have to tell them the truth about his hidden life and his diagnosis.

"What if they reject me?" he asked.

"That is always a possibility," I said. "Having them come is not without risk. But, if you choose not to have them come, you take the risk of missing a great deal of support they could offer."

Ray decided to take the risk, and I made the phone call to let them know he wanted to see them. Ray felt close to Bob and Doris because he had worked in the bank with his brother as a teenager and had lived in their home. They came and spent the weekend. Ray told them who he was and what was happening. They were shocked almost beyond words but were gracious despite the shock. Before they left, Bob took my hand and said, "If you ever need anything, just let me know." It was a shining moment in the darkness.

5

The Battle
for Ray's Body

We rode the AIDS roller coaster week after week, and other members of Ray's immediate family visited on weekends until all three brothers and his sister had spent time with him and heard his story. Each time I sat with him on the bed, and he held my hand tightly under the covers while he recounted the events leading up to his diagnosis of AIDS. The emotional stress was exhausting.

The unreal quality of my life continued. It all seemed like a nightmare. I was confused and asked myself, Who was I to Ray? A friend, his wife, the mother of his children, companion, his housekeeper? Certainly not his lover. I could not understand how he could have carried on his other relationships and then come home and be my husband. What a sham!

As the weeks churned along, it became clear that the virus was winning. Although my siblings and my mother knew Ray was ill, they had not been told the diagnosis. It was time to tell them and invite them to visit. My three siblings came from northern Indiana. (My mother was in a nursing home and did not come.) Although all were shocked, they were caring, considering the brief time they had to adjust to the unexpected events.

Ray had changed in significant ways, yet much remained the same. He complained of almost every aspect of his care. He criticized his nurses, the lab and X-ray technicians, housekeepers, and the dietary department. No one could please him except his primary physicians. His nurses dreaded coming into his room because of his complaints. I understood that it is not unusual for terminally people to vent their frustrations on those who care for them, but that did not make it easier for those who became his targets.

He made little effort to do for himself things he could do. Drinking adequate fluids was of great importance. I brought fresh mint tea regularly because he did not like the water. Ice was easily available, so he could have had fresh iced tea any time. At first he was glad to have a choice and drank more, but after a few days he did not bother to ask for ice or reach for the tea. Early in July he almost died of renal failure because of dehydration. He showed little interest in living.

"Ray, you have to *fight* this disease," I said.

"Why? Just so another infection can come along and take me?"

Several of his friends had already died of AIDS-related infections, so he was not motivated to help himself. Later, as I learned more about a compromised immune system and saw many people with AIDS, I understood his attitude much better.

In the end I was thankful he did not suffer longer. He lived only seven weeks and two days after his diagnosis, the day of truth. There were times during those weeks when it seemed he had been ill forever and other times when I could scarcely endure knowing that his time was going to be so short. I often felt numb. My emotions were supersaturated. I talked about Ray and his illness, even his impending death, with unbelievable objectivity. I was so tired physically I sometimes wished the end would come soon. What would life be like without him? I wondered. On the heels of such thoughts came the awareness that when his life was over, our life together would be over forever.

The loving support of good friends, the concern of people in our church, Scripture, prayer, and music nurtured me and gave me strength to live each day. A Gospel passage in John 11:4 became living truth for me one morning. "This illness does not lead to death; rather it is for God's glory, so that the Son of God may be glorified through it." Not for a moment did I think this meant Ray would regain his physical health. However, I became confident that his life and suffering were not to be in vain. I felt reassured that in some way God would use what was happening to bring something positive from it if I remained open to that possibility.

My dear friend, Marie, came to our home one evening. She knew Ray was ill but wanted to hear what his illness meant for me. The memory of her visit has been an enduring gift. She was a chaplain in one of the Chicago area medical centers and often sang and played her guitar for her patients. I asked if she would consider singing for Ray and me. She graciously agreed, and we set a time for her to come to the hospital. Her visit was like an oasis in the desert of illness. She sang song after song as Ray and I listened and wept together. The song I treasured above all others, "Be Not Afraid," is based on Isaiah 43:2-3. I listened to a recording of it all summer long.

> You shall cross the barren desert, but you shall not
>   die of thirst.
> You shall wander far in safety though you do not
>   know the way.
> You shall speak your words in foreign lands and all
>   will understand.
> They shall see the face of God and live.
>
> *Chorus:*
> Be not afraid, I go before you always,
> Come, follow me, and I will give you rest.

Verse 2:
When you pass through raging waters, in the sea
you shall not drown,
When you walk amid the burning flames, you shall
not be harmed,
If you stand before the powers of hell, and death is at
your side,
Know that I am with you through it all.

Text copyright © 1975, 1978 Robert J. Dufford, SJ, and New Dawn Music. Published by OCP Publications, 5536 NE Hessalo, Portland, OR 97213

We were refreshed and renewed by her music.

On the last Sunday in July two special friends, Marcus and Dottie, came from Elkhart, Indiana, to visit. Marcus had been our pastor in Oregon from 1963–1966. Over lunch the three of us reminisced about those important Oregon years. I updated them on the course of events, beginning with the early symptoms I had noticed the previous fall, up to the current situation. It was good preparation for them to relate to Ray with acceptance, understanding, and compassion. When we arrived at the hospital, Dottie, a nurse, sat at the bedside while Ray clung to her hand for the entire visit. The fact that Marcus earlier had been our pastor was especially healing for all of us.

The next day, when I arrived at the hospital around noon, I stopped at the nurse's station and asked, "How is Ray doing this morning?"

"It's hard to tell. He didn't have much to say this morning while I bathed him and changed the bed linens. Why don't you go talk to him and see what you think?" I recognized the nurse's remarks as a gentle warning. I needed only a few minutes at the bedside to understand why she had said what she did. Ray's eyes were open but vacant and staring straight ahead. He appeared to be unaware of my presence until I called his name to catch his attention. His responses were brief and he initiated no conversation. He was obviously weak, his condition having deteriorated substantially since the previous afternoon.

Before going home for a short rest, I told his nurse I wanted to visit with Dr. Moore when he came to see his patients later that evening. My intention was to return to the hospital soon. As it turned out I had several unexpected delays and did not get back to the hospital until around eight that evening.

The nurse in charge greeted me: "Dr. Moore has been waiting three hours for you." I was appalled. "I didn't mean for him to wait for me," I said, chagrined. It was highly unusual in my experience for a doctor to wait in the hospital for the return of a family member. Leaving a telephone number where he or she could be reached, yes, but to actually wait for a family member, never.

"He is waiting for you in the conference room," said the nurse.

"I'm sorry, Dr. Moore," I said. "I didn't mean for you to wait."

"We need to talk and I didn't want to do it by phone. The virus has invaded the brain. That's why he is less alert and doesn't speak readily. Would you be willing to give permission for an autopsy?"

"If it could provide clues useful in treating others, I have no objections." I signed the necessary forms. I appreciated that Dr. Moore chose not to discuss such a difficult matter over the phone. I knew he could have left the forms with the nurses and asked one of them to get permission from me; instead he chose to speak with me face-to-face. Such sensitivity provided much needed trust amid the chaos and relentless movement toward Ray's final days.

After those first horrible days, when the medical resident asked me to leave the room, I was always treated with the greatest respect and courtesy by Dr. Moore and Dr. Blatt. They were partners in medical practice as well as partners in life. I also realized the resident had been following Ray's wishes.

As soon as Ray had given his illness a name and told me his physicians were gay men, I understood the reasons for his secrecy before and during the early days of his hospitalization. Dr. Moore later told me he and Ray "had words" the day Ray went for the biopsy report. The doctor had tried his best to persuade Ray to be honest with me, but to no avail. Ray didn't know what the doctors would find, but he had been terrified. He was also terrified I would leave him once I knew he had been sexually active outside our marriage. Once the diagnosis was definitive, it was his friend Bill who convinced him to take the risk of being truthful with me. It was apparent that nothing short of what happened would have motivated Ray to risk telling me the truth earlier.

In the later years of our marriage, I had often prayed that God would allow whatever was needed to come into Ray's life to open him and bring him healing. I certainly do not believe God *punished* Ray with AIDS. What seems much more likely to me is that, in giving me that prayer, God had been preparing me to accept whatever would come our way.

6

August 1984

The Long Watch

Wednesday morning, August 1, I was at the hospital early to see Dr. Moore when he made his morning rounds. After checking Ray's condition, he nodded for me to follow him into the hallway. "There is one more lab report I want to see, but I think the time probably has come for you to take Ray home." (I had told Dr. Moore earlier that, when nothing more could be done for Ray in the hospital, both of us wanted him to come home to die.)

Dr. Moore returned within a few minutes. "There is really nothing more we can do for him here. You may take him home."

"All right, I'll take him tomorrow."

"If he lives that long."

"You mean he might not?" My voice was tense, higher pitched than usual.

"He may have twelve hours, twenty-four at the most." Dr. Moore spoke softly but firmly.

"Then I'll take him home today."

Within minutes a nurse was at the bedside. She asked, "Ray would you like to go home?"

He nodded. He appeared more alert almost immediately, yet extremely weak. The staff helped me pack his belongings, and I carried them to the car in a daze. Ray was to be transported home by ambulance later. I had a few hours to prepare our bedroom for him.

Once at home, I called a young couple from our church who had volunteered to help with whatever we needed. "Ray is coming home this afternoon to die. Will you please arrange for someone to be with me around the clock to help with his care? He requires total care. It isn't possible to manage alone." They agreed to make the arrangements.

I called our daughter Karen in Kansas. "If you want to see your father once more while he is alive, you need to come as quickly as possible. He is coming home from the hospital this afternoon." I knew she would be on her way without delay.

Soon an oxygen machine was delivered. It was the only mechanical device to be used. It would ease his breathing. Our primary concern at this point was to keep Ray as comfortable as possible. The ambulance arrived with him in mid-afternoon, and the attendants carefully put him into bed. His whole body was highly sensitive to touch, needing to be moved carefully to avoid pain. He was little more than skin and bone. He had aged twenty-five years during his eight weeks in the hospital.

I thought he needed some kind of nourishment and mixed a small milkshake for him. As I approached the bed, he lifted both hands to signal no. He sipped iced tea through a straw until he became too weak, then I switched to a teaspoon and finally to a medicine dropper to help keep him hydrated.

The first two helpers from the church arrived in late afternoon. Ray was too weak to say more than a few words at a time but recognized everyone. All who came were aware of the diagnosis yet tenderly assisted with his care. They came for two- to four-hour shifts, usually two people together.

The next day, Thursday, was memorable for several reasons. Dr. Moore came to the house Thursday forenoon to see how we were getting along. That meant a fifty-minute drive through the city each way. I was astonished once more by his kindness and care; I thought the days when doctors made house calls were long gone.

A day or so before Ray came home, his address book had been open on his bedside table though I had not seen it there earlier. I noticed the name of a man I will call Frank. On Thursday forenoon, I opened the apartment door in answer to a knock. A neatly dressed stranger greeted me.

"Hello, my name is Frank. I am a friend of Ray's. I went to the hospital to see him and was told he had been discharged. May I see him?"

There had been so many surprises during the past eight weeks that not much flustered me anymore.

"Just a minute, let me check with Ray." I went to the bedroom and said quietly, "Ray, Frank is at the door to see you. Shall I invite him in?" A look of painful distress crossed his face. He remained silent.

I returned to the door, invited Frank into the living room, and offered him a seat. "A painful expression crossed Ray's face when I told him you were here. I don't think it is wise for you to go see him." Frank made no objection and asked no questions. I sat down to chat with him for a few minutes.

"I cared about Ray a great deal and wanted him to move in with me, but he refused because he didn't want to leave you. After everything is over I'd like to have lunch with you sometime." My head was spinning when he left.

Karen arrived from Kansas that afternoon, carrying a handful of wild sunflowers she had picked on her way to Kansas City to catch her plane. She knew how much Ray loved wild sunflowers. He was still conscious and pleased to see her and to receive her gift.

Krista, initially hurt and angry when Ray told his story, wrote a compassionate letter that I read to him. I was happy it had arrived while he was still conscious. It was an important step in bringing closure to her relationship with her father—a beautiful gift to him and her.

The most dramatic and treasured story of the day occurred early that evening around Ray's bed. We noticed his breathing becoming shallow and slow. We thought that death was only minutes away. I called our friend, Bob. He arrived shortly since he lived nearby. He greeted Ray, then sat at the bedside to read a portion of Scripture and pray. When he began the Lord's Prayer, Ray joined him until his strength was gone. Everything was quiet for a few moments after the prayer. Suddenly Ray's eyes opened wide. The vacant look was gone. He was alert, totally present. He smiled at us and shook his fist playfully as he made a joke. The moment was awesome, sacred. We had witnessed an epiphany, God's presence. It was a gift beyond price that will endure forever, even though it lasted less than a minute before he lapsed back into his weakened state. His breathing was more normal again. At last, Ray's inner child, his lively little boy, had come out to play, and I knew he was healed of his inner conflict.

Early Friday morning a similar episode occurred. Ray's breathing slowed and became shallow. I called Bob. He came, read Scripture, and prayed with us. Momentarily Ray's eyes cleared, and he was alert and present. However, this time Karen and I were the sole focus of his attention. It was as if we were the only people in the room. We watched in breathless wonder.

By afternoon Ray could no longer swallow. He kept his hand on his forehead much of the time. His body burned with fever.

"Is your head hurting?" I asked. He nodded. The doctor had left medication for severe pain, but I wanted a nurse to administer it. One from our congregation arrived to take her turn early that evening. I told her Ray's head had been hurting for several hours. "The doctor left suppositories for pain, but I wanted you to administer one of them."

"I can do that as long as you are aware he will probably become comatose and may not regain consciousness again if we use it."

"It is more important to me that he is comfortable than that he is conscious," I said. She gave him the medication. He slipped into unconsciousness within a short time and rested much more easily.

I felt torn. I was ready for the long watch to be over, but I realized that with his last breath, his life on earth would be over forever. I had a profound sense of the finality of death. No matter how much I had prepared for the moment, I was ambivalent as the time approached.

Dr. Moore called on Saturday morning, "What is happening? Is Ray still with us?"

"He is still with us," I said.

"I can't imagine what is keeping him alive."

"One of our chaplain friends said he is alive because he is soaking up all the love that surrounds him."

"That must be it. There is *nothing* else to keep him alive."

On Saturday afternoon a nurse gave Ray additional medication for pain, since he had become restless. I lay in our bed beside him, singing softly to him as I stroked his chest. We kept cool, wet towels on his chest to ease his raging fever.

A young medical student who attended our church came late Saturday evening to help with Ray's care. Sam kept watch with Karen as she held her father's hand, while I caught a short nap. I had asked Sam to awaken me in time to be with Ray at the end. He promised to do that. A few minutes after 1:00 a.m. on Sunday, Sam came into the living room and awakened me. "It won't be long now," he said. Karen was still holding her father's hand, and Sam and I stood at the bedside as Ray drew his last few breaths. The long watch was over.

Instead of living twelve hours, Ray had lived more than three and a half days, over eighty hours! Those days had been intense in every conceivable way, yet I cannot think of anything in all the world I would give in exchange for our time together.

Sam was on hand to call the mortuary to come for the body and to notify Dr. Moore that Ray had died. He stayed the rest of the night and prepared breakfast for us before notifying the people from our church. When Sue heard that Ray had died, she said, "Ann won't feel like coming to church this morning. Why don't we go to her house for church?" So on Sunday morning we celebrated worship in our living room. I was truly blessed. To have Karen present and to be surrounded by our church family was to know that I was loved.

None of us that morning could have guessed how deeply the experience of caring for Ray during the last days of his life would change our congregation in the future. The transforming power of that experience will become apparent later.

I was like Nicodemus: "How can these things be?" (John 3:9). In a mysterious way, as I had continued my journey with Ray into the center of our pain, I realized that salvation, grace, redemption, forgiveness, suffering, death, and resurrection had become our lived experience. All these realities were so intertwined that I could not have separated any one dimension from the rest. As I entered fully into my pain instead of resisting or turning from it, I discovered God was present *in* the pain, redeeming and healing all. We were not alone. The One who had created me, created Ray, had joined us in our suffering.

Surely God did not abandon Ray even while he was living a double life and Ray had not abandoned God. Had he been conscious of God's presence during that time? Do the barriers we erect between each other also become barriers that keep us from experiencing God's presence? Often when I felt distant from Ray I also felt distant from God. It became essential that I had at least a few people to whom I related closely for me to be aware of God's presence. There is so much about life to contemplate.

7

The Unfinished Lives

Dear Ray,
You won my heart years ago,
now you left me
with life unfinished—
yours and mine.
So briefly we tasted new joy,
closeness—
the barriers gone,
breathing the sweet fresh
air of truth.
The memories of the
last seven weeks
sparkle like rare jewels
crafted in the fires
of our suffering.
You had only a sip of the
wine of freedom from
the fear of discovery.
The cost of your secret
so high!
I'm so sad, so sad
our children no longer

have a father.
One whom they cherish,
whose love they crave.
Your grandchildren will
never know you
nor you them.
You know nothing of their
achievements or
disappointments and pain.
Your death leaves us with
so much unfinished,
so much searching
and growing to do,
the journey formidable.
So many questions
unanswered—
many people to know,
so much grieving and
healing to pursue.
Ray, years ago you won my heart.
Now you left me
with life unfinished—
yours and mine.
I will persevere!

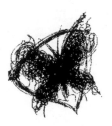

Part Two

O LORD, you have searched me and known me.
You know when I sit down and when I rise up;
you discern my thoughts from far away.
You search out my path and my lying down,
and are acquainted with all my ways.
Even before a word is on my tongue,
O LORD, you know it completely.
You hem me in, behind and before,
and lay your hand upon me.
Such knowledge is too wonderful for me;
it is so high that I cannot attain it.
Where can I go from your spirit?
Or where can I flee from your presence?
If I ascend to heaven, you are there;
if I make my bed in Sheol, you are there.
If I take the wings of the morning
and settle at the farthest limits of the sea,
even there your hand shall lead me,
and your right hand shall hold me fast.
—Psalm 139:1-10

8

Setting the Stage

Earlier I referred to "a long story." Part two consists of that story and provides the background for understanding the other three parts of the book. To understand the long story it is important to consider the radical differences between the world Ray and I knew growing up and the world we lived in at the time Ray revealed his diagnosis and his hidden life as a gay man.

Ray and I grew up in families that had little experience in expressing feelings, whether of tenderness or of disappointment, fear or anger. Children were to be seen, not heard. Discipline was strict and the subject of sex was taboo. (Although I was raised on a farm until age sixteen, I had never seen an animal being born. That was strictly the men's domain.) Difficulties or conflicts in the family were endured stoically or hidden as much as possible. Such rigid controls may have been exaggerated in our families but were not foreign to many people in society at large.

Many women began working outside the home during World War II, and some of them did not return to the kitchen when the war was over. Women seeking careers in addition to family responsibilities became more common. The major changes that followed during the 1960s and 1970s—the civil rights movement, the feminist movement, the sexual revolution, the Vietnam war, and the "coming out" of the gay community—combined to create such enormous upheavals in society that no one was left untouched and no institutions unchanged. The time when many would speak easily of regularly consulting their therapist was still in the distant future. Nothing had prepared us for the complexity of our gay/straight marriage.

9

1929–1950

The Early Years—Ray[1]

My perception of Ray's early life has been developed from the stories he told me before and after we were married. More recently his sister added to the picture and refreshed the earlier memories.

Ray's father, grandparents, and several aunts and uncles moved to the plains of south-central Kansas from the beautiful Shenandoah Valley of Virginia in the early years of the twentieth century. Ray's father was a farmer and taught school before going into banking, the business he pursued the rest of his working years.

At the time of Ray's birth the family lived in the small town of Yoder, Kansas. His father owned the Farmers State Bank in Yoder. Ray was the youngest of four boys and one girl. He was born in 1929, on the eve of the Great Depression. His sister, closest to him in age, remembers going with her father to the hospital to see and hold her new brother while sitting on the bed with their mother. She was also permitted to choose the baby's name to compensate for the keen disappointment she felt in not getting the sister she so wanted.

Ray always told me that when he began working in the bank, he needed to stand on a low stool to see over the counter while serving customers. He was good in math and later was meticulous in keeping account of our finances. Every penny had to be accounted for when he reconciled the bank statement.

The family lived simply and frugally. Their house was so small the three older boys slept in a back room of the bank, located a stone's throw from the house. That is, they slept there until the night several robbers crept through the room where they were sleeping on their way to torch the vault to carry off the money. After that the three slept on the floor at home until a large room could be prepared for them in the basement.

Ray's parents attended the Yoder Mennonite Church, a mile north of town. He was baptized and became a member of the church at age eleven or twelve. He maintained at least marginal connection with his home congregation through occasional participation in youth activities until he left the community as a young adult.

Ray began his education at Harmony, a two-room school, in Yoder. Grades one through four were in one room and grades five through eight in the other. Later he left home to live with his grandmother and one of his aunts after his grandfather's death. He was ready for the eighth grade when he moved in with his grandmother and attended school in that community.

Like many Mennonite young people in the area, Ray attended high school in the academy located on the campus of Hesston College, a Mennonite junior college in Hesston, Kansas. He completed the spring semester of his senior year of high school by correspondence and worked with his oldest brother in the bank in Yoder. He lived with his brother and sister-in-law because his parents had moved to Buhler, another small Kansas town, where his father owned another bank. Ray had completed his correspondence course in time to graduate with his class at Hesston in June 1947.

The Mennonite church began providing opportunities for young people to volunteer in various summer projects in the mid-1940s. In 1947 they opened the first long-term (one-year) service unit in Kansas City, Missouri. The volunteers lived together in a house with houseparents and worked as orderlies and nurses' aides in Kansas City General Hospital, a large charity hospital nearby. Except for a small stipend, the volunteers contributed their earnings to run the household and to support the larger voluntary service program.

Ray decided to join the Kansas City unit when it opened. He had no previous experience in hospitals but considered it an adventure. He found the hospital work interesting and challenging. The following year he moved to Hannibal, Missouri, and again chose to work as an orderly in a hospital and kept his earnings. In summer 1950, he joined a group of Mennonite young people who went to Europe for ten weeks under the auspices of Mennonite Central Committee. They were engaged in volunteer work in war-ravaged areas for four weeks, then traveled for six weeks. Ray returned to Kansas just in time to enroll at Hesston College for his freshman year. The two years he spent working in hospitals had piqued his interest in the nursing profession.

10

1930–1943

The Early Years—Ann

The kerosene lamp shed a dim circle of light in the bedroom. The family doctor, along with my father, Jacob, and Tillie, the "hired girl"—as household help was known among the Amish—attended my mother as she gave birth. The hands of the clock pointed to a few minutes before midnight on that bitterly cold January night when they heard my first cry. I had arrived in time to be a birthday gift for my mother, the youngest of seven children, born into an Old Order Amish family. We were four boys and three girls. Several years after my birth, my maternal grandparents, Dan and Mattie, arrived to share our home and complete a three-generation household of eleven. My oldest brother, Samuel, was twelve when I was born. John was eleven, my sister Tillie nine, Clarence was eight, Elizabeth six, and Aden not yet five.

A delightful memory of sitting with Aden in a rocker in front of the pot-bellied stove lingers in my mind. We often sat in the rocker singing a song about a shoemaker and watching the dancing flames through the little isinglass rectangles in the stove door. Mouth-watering aromas of ham and biscuits emanating from the kitchen added a sense of coziness and safety.

I often played by myself as a young child since all the rest were in school by the time of my earliest memory. With a lively imagination, I frequently created playmates until I discovered that creating an imaginary reality was not acceptable. My mother was not pleased with my creative activity. Why would you want to pretend something that is not "real"? Why entertain thoughts that are not "true"? Later I learned that reading fiction was frowned upon for the same reason. Only factual truth was to be trusted. There was no room for the figurative or the mythical or the imaginary. Mother's concern was always, Why would you want to read or write what is not "true"?

What a great loss! Listening to a story in preaching class during my senior year in seminary, I began to reclaim my imagination, making it possible for me to enter the biblical stories in a much deeper, more personal way and thereby gain fresh insights and a greater understanding of the text.

A little white clapboard house set in a small farmyard at the end of a long lane was home. South of the house was the outhouse (a two-holer), the garden, and a field between the house and the gravel road. To the east were the chicken house, the round brooder house, and a small orchard. The barn where we milked the cows and kept the horses stood to the north side of the farmyard. The barn, once painted red, long ago had exchanged its brightness for the dull gray of well-weathered siding, silent testimony to years of rain, sleet, snow, and the bone-chilling winter winds of central Indiana.

Farm horses are wonderful animals—huge, tame, sleek, and strong. I liked the horses. The pigs poked their noses into the feeding trough and under the fence somewhere else in the farmyard. Since I had little to do with them, I don't recall their location. Oh, but I do remember the little piglets lying in a tight row, nuzzling up to mama pig's "milk-factory outlet," gulping down their milk. If there happened to be a runt in the litter, Dad would bring it into the house in a basket and place it on the open oven door in the kitchen to keep the piglet warm.

Occasionally we had to bottle feed the little runt for a few days until it was strong enough to fend for itself.

Our farm was small, only thirty-five acres. Dad farmed with horses and also worked a neighbor's farm on a crop-sharing basis to increase the family income. Dad lived and worked with the intensity of a man who felt the welfare of the world depended on him. Indeed, the welfare of his world—his large family—did depend on him and on Mother, Lovina. The daily presence of my grandparents was a living reminder of what could happen if taxes and the mortgage payments were not met.

"Everyone works at our house" was a well-known and oft-repeated phrase around the farm. It was true. We were all assigned our share of chores at an early age. Dad, for reasons I never understood, enjoyed taking care of the chickens. The chickens were fine but I disliked the smell of the chicken house. One of my early tasks was to follow Dad around to gather the eggs. Later I was expected to keep Mom supplied with dry corncobs that she used for starting the fire in the kitchen stove. Keeping the wood-box filled was next on the list and finally learning to milk a cow. I progressed to milking before I started school at age seven. Learning to take responsibility and doing good work is a legacy I have long appreciated.

Discipline in the family was stiff. My parents took literally the admonition in Proverbs 22:15: "Folly is bound up in the heart of a [child], but the rod of discipline drives it far away." The "rod" fell severely and often. Dad's word was law and Mother supported him.

However, a day came when one of the boys, while being whipped by Mom, didn't make a sound. Since he was silent, she beat harder and harder. When she finally stopped, he turned to her and in a voice filled with rage asked, "Are you through?" Every movement of his body shouted his rage as he strode to the door of the washhouse, slamming the door as if to tear it from its hinges. His message apparently reached a place in Mom's heart that screams of pain and tears had not reached. She was frightened. Behind the scenes Mom appealed to Dad to change their method of discipline. She realized corporal punishment was not accomplishing what she and Dad intended.

Although they had modified the frequency of severe punishment by the time I was growing up, it did not stop. I remember seething with anger after being punished in a way that left painfully stinging welts on my back. I sometimes went to a safe place to nurse my anger and think, *Someday it will be my turn*, or *Just wait, I'll show them*. I'm no longer sure what "showing them" meant except to bring a measure of comfort and, in a way I could not have articulated, to provide a glimmer of hope for a future when I would make my own decisions.

Now, so many years later, I wonder: could those thoughts have been whispers of the Spirit protecting me from complete despair? Amid my grief after Ray's death, a phrase from Psalm 4:1 became a living word to me: "Answer me when I call, O God of my right! *You gave me room when I was in distress*" (my emphasis). Is it possible that God was giving me room in my distress when I was a young child, helpless in the face of such harsh discipline?

My parents, like so many people during the Great Depression, were very poor. Yet we were fortunate because most of our food came from the farm. There was always a large vegetable garden from which we harvested and canned hundreds of quarts of food each summer. Meat, milk, and eggs were produced on the farm as well. However, there was almost no cash to buy staples such as flour, sugar, and salt, or to buy shoes and cloth for the clothes Mom sewed for her growing children. Two stories of desperate need and of the unusual ways in which they were met will remain with me throughout life.

Property taxes would be due within a few months. There was no cash. The very real possibility of losing the farm confronted Mom and Dad. There were a few acres of alfalfa that Dad cut for hay in the spring. After the first cutting, he decided not to cut the second growth but to harvest the seed later. Harvest time arrived. The alfalfa was cut and threshed. The crop yielded more seed per acre than any Dad ever had harvested. The man who threshed it said he had never seen such a large yield from so small an acreage. Dad sold the seed for the amount needed to pay the taxes. My parents celebrated with a thanksgiving fast. That's right: a fast, not a feast. The feast was the abundant crop that had supplied their urgent need.

A second story: The flour supply was almost gone and there was no money to buy more. Dad was on his way to town on business. He was burdened by the dilemma he faced. What was he to do? How would he feed the family? His thoughts were a prayer. Later, as he walked down Main Street, he passed a store with a huge bag of flour in the front window. Beside it was a sign advertising a contest. The person who came closest to guessing the number of pounds of flour would win the whole bag. Dad looked at the bag for a long time, estimating the number of twenty-five-pound bags that would fit into the larger sack. He went inside and submitted his estimate. Several days later he was notified that he had won. Two hundred twenty-five pounds of flour were his! Dad never doubted that wisdom beyond his own guided him in making his estimate.

Mom and Dad were very devout. As a young man Dad had lived in Oregon for several years. There was no Amish community where he lived and worked, so he chose to attend services with an Evangelical United Brethren congregation. There he experienced a life-changing conversion of the heart. Dad was a reader and became thoroughly acquainted with the Bible. He was able to turn immediately to almost any Scripture on any subject.

Dad saw no reason to leave the Amish church following his conversion. Instead he determined to contribute to a deeper spiritual life from within the church. That decision led him to listen to the inner direction of his own heart and spirit rather than depending on the church leaders for his only or even his primary spiritual understanding. Dad often disagreed with the church leaders and was not diplomatic in stating his views. In fact, he could be downright dogmatic.

After returning to Indiana from Oregon, he courted and married Lovina, who became my mother. His serious ambition was to raise a model family, children in whom he would instill knowledge of the Scriptures and teach strict obedience. He hoped that his family would influence other people in the Amish church to greater spiritual exploration and commitment. I have never questioned the sincerity of Dad's ambition but feel compelled to ask how his goal may have affected his choice of discipline, to say nothing about the wisdom of such a goal.

Every morning after breakfast, we pushed away from the table and moved into the living room for family worship. Mom and Dad read alternately through a chapter from the German Bible. Even though I did not understand every word, I understood much of it. All Scripture read in our church services were also in German, and we spoke a German dialect in the family. Mom and Dad read the Psalms, the creation narratives, the stories of Noah, the patriarchs, Moses, David, and many more. They read the New Testament Gospels and Epistles, but the readings that I found both fascinating and frightening were those from the Revelation of St. John. The images of strange beasts with multiple heads and horns, the threat of hailstones, mountains falling, and pits of fire and brimstone scared me terribly. After the reading we all knelt as Dad read from his German prayer book.

In the evening at bedtime, the family gathered once more and knelt together for evening prayer. Our life was lived within this framework of morning worship and evening prayer. The faith of my parents as expressed in the complete consistency of this rhythm of worship and work is alive at the center of my being as an anchor that has held me through all the vicissitudes of life. There was never a question in my mind what they considered more important, work or worship. I bless them for their gift.

Dad insisted that we conform to all the external rules of the Amish church concerning dress codes and forgoing modern conveniences. At the same time he made it clear to us that he did not regard such externals as essential to the heart of the gospel message. It was not unusual for him to take the family to special services—conferences or revival meetings—at the local Mennonite church. In our community that was not forbidden although at the time few Amish people chose to attend such meetings. Often revival preaching included frequent references to hellfire and the danger of delaying "getting right" with God. It was a frightening prospect for a young child with a tender heart.

The severe punishment combined with revival preaching created intense guilt, haunting fear, and a pervasive sense of worthlessness by the time I was eleven or twelve. Furthermore, my Dad's insistence that we conform to all the external rules of the church while at the same time making it clear he did not think of them as central to faith felt like a mixed message and added to the confusion to my inner life. My parents would have been bewildered and distressed had they known the degree of anxiety and inner conflict that troubled me in late childhood.

My mother was plagued with serious episodes of depression soon after the birth of her fourth child. Since I was the youngest of the seven children, the dense gloom that settled over the whole family when Mom was depressed was a complete mystery to me for many years.

When Mom was depressed, Dad did not whistle as he went about his early morning chores the way he usually did. His telltale silence was almost deafening. "Don't talk, don't have fun, don't even smile, Mom isn't feeling well," his silence shouted. No word of explanation was ever given to help us understand the dramatic change of mood that occurred periodically. How *could* our parents acknowledge the reality? In the early years of the twentieth century, emotional problems were considered shameful, a sign of weakness, often understood as a lack of faith by religious people. Mom and Dad suffered in silence until the episode passed, just as we children suffered.

My oldest sister, Tillie, became a surrogate mother to me in my early years. We had few books in the house, but Tillie had saved her pennies until she finally had enough money to purchase a Bible in English. She often told a Bible story in bed before we fell asleep, all three girls in one bed. For some reason the story of the man on the cross usually evoked feelings of sadness and pity.

11

1944–1949

Adolescence to Young Adulthood—Ann

Tillie left home when she was twenty-one and went to Virginia, where her favorite aunt lived. She left the Old Order Church soon after leaving home. When I was fourteen she wrote a letter that changed my life. She wondered if I might be searching to know how to become a Christian as she had searched earlier. She suggested I read two passages of Scripture and accept them as if meant for me personally. The first, Romans 10:9—10, reads as follows: "if you confess with your lips that Jesus is Lord and believe in your heart that God raised him from the dead, you will be saved. For one believes with the heart and so is justified, and one confesses with the mouth and so is saved." The second passage is found in 1 John 1:9: "If we confess our sins, he who is faithful and just will forgive us our sins and cleanse us from all unrighteousness." I read the passages, knelt beside my bed, and prayed a very simple prayer confessing myself a sinner and Jesus Christ as Savior; I promised to serve God all my life. It was a serious commitment to make before God at fourteen years of age.

How does one describe what is indescribable? Today, after sixty years, I still search for words that communicate what happened as I prayed that simple prayer. The best I can do is to say it was like a dark room suddenly filled with brilliant light, joy, and peace. I said nothing to anyone about the experience for a long time. Even though my parents were devout, we did not speak to each other about personal faith. Why I didn't write and tell my sister what had happened, I will never know, but I didn't.

My parents knew something unusual had occurred because of the way I went about my daily duties. Joy instead of complaint spoke for itself. The euphoria lasted for about a week. Then I began to obsess about the possibility that I might have failed in some way to "please" God during that week. What if I had not kept my promise to serve God? What if I had lied to God? I moved from joy to fear and torment. I began to read my Bible hungrily, searching for something that would bring back the joy and peace I had felt. There were short periods when I did find peace, but there was also great confusion as I tried desperately to be "good enough."

Since I had been taught that all of Scripture is God's Word, I took everything I read with great seriousness. My father was highly suspicious of Bible commentaries and there were certainly none in our home. He wanted us to "think for our selves"—as long as our thoughts agreed with his! So I muddled my way through the confusion. Later several of my siblings and I once again attended a revival meeting at the local Mennonite church. I went forward for prayer when the altar call was given. I no longer remember the details of the prayers. What I do remember is that before I had the opportunity to do so, one of my siblings told my parents I had gone forward for prayer. Mother asked several days later what my going forward meant and what I was going to do about it. "If I would be staying at home this winter, I would join the Mennonite church," I responded. Nothing more was said.

I was a freshman in high school at the time all of the above was happening, and attending high school was not looked upon with favor by leaders in the Amish church. My parents were planning to go to Florida for the winter months and asked if I wanted to go along. It seemed like a good opportunity. I dropped out of school and went along. Liz, my sister, seven years older than I, went along as well. Mom and Dad rented a small house in a village that was a winter home for many Amish and Mennonite people. Going to Florida for the winter was not a vacation for my parents; it was a place where Dad could work all winter long. He had health problems during the severe winters of central Indiana.

Our parents sometimes attended the Amish church service but also frequented the Mennonite church. Liz and I always went to the Mennonite church. The most significant event of that winter was my baptism. Liz found out through a friend that the bishop with oversight of the Mennonite congregations in Florida was in the area for a few weeks. He was planning a baptismal service during his stay. Liz and I decided to visit the bishop on a Saturday afternoon to ask if he would baptize me. Although we were complete strangers, he received us graciously. I told him of my desire to be baptized though I had never received any formal instruction for baptism. I indicated my willingness to receive instruction afterward. He assured me there was no problem. He asked no questions about my parents or whether they knew about my plans. Nothing! Today, as a minister, it is difficult for me to imagine such unquestioning readiness to baptize a fifteen-year-old and a complete stranger.

It was time to go home and tell my parents. The news took them completely by surprise. They were hurt that I had not asked them before making the arrangements with the bishop. Despite their hurt, they were not going to "stand in my way." Knowing I had hurt my parents left me feeling guilty and robbed me of the joy I had anticipated. I had chosen not to speak with them before going to see the bishop because I knew if they voiced any objections, I would not have the courage to oppose their wishes. It was a difficult dilemma because I felt I had to follow what I understood to be the God-given desire of my heart.

The next several years were a period of intense spiritual and emotional anguish. The move from one faith tradition to another was a difficult journey for me. Virtually everything related to the Amish way of life had religious significance. That was true whether it had to do with the color of shoes or hose, plain versus print fabric for the clothes we wore, the proper length for dresses, short or long sleeves, the particular style of prayer covering, on and on. For someone with a desperate desire to "measure up," to be "good enough" to be "pleasing to God," a need to sort through the minutiae to determine what had true significance for faith in and commitment to Christ was a formidable task.

Emotionally I was severely depressed and withdrew into myself. I rarely initiated conversation with anyone whom I did not know well. My parents sensed something was wrong but had no idea how to respond.

My sister Tillie in her mid-twenties returned home for a visit the summer I was sixteen. She soon realized I was in trouble emotionally. She suggested to my parents that it was important for me to leave home. Her plan was that I go with her to Hesston, Kansas, where she planned to return for her second year of college. (I was unaware of this discussion for many years.) Since I had never returned to high school following my winter in Florida, the opportunity to go to Hesston to attend the academy seemed like a good option. I was permitted to room with Tillie even though she lived in the dormitory for the college girls. I'm not sure I could have adjusted to living with a stranger at that point.

I had always enjoyed school and did well in my studies. The same was true at Hesston. But finding my way socially was difficult because of my reluctance to initiate any kind of social interaction. Not surprisingly, my depression followed me to Hesston though I didn't even know the word except as it applied to a time when our family was extremely poor. Often when I was depressed and not speaking to anyone, Tillie demanded that I talk to her. She simply outwaited me, no matter how long it took for me to express what was troubling me. There is no way to know what would have happened to me without a sister who truly cared. Her concern and support held me steady when I was afraid of losing my moorings. Little by little I began to emerge from my shell and to develop friendships with others, like the tiny bud of a flower opening ever so slowly to sunshine, fresh air, and rain.

It was encouraging to meet fellow students who were serious about faith yet knew how to enjoy life. Many students as well as faculty members were outgoing, friendly people. Enrollment was small enough that most of us knew everyone else by name. The atmosphere on campus was congenial and conducive to personal growth. By the close of the school year, there was no question about my wanting to return the following year even though Tillie was graduating with a diploma from both the academy and the junior college.

My parents had moved to Ohio in the fall of 1946, the year Tillie and I lived in Kansas. They decided that moving into a new community was a good time for them to leave the Amish church. What a transition! To have seen five of their seven children leave the Amish church had made a deep impact on Mom and Dad. It is to their credit they were able embrace their own deeper understanding of faith and to become part of a Mennonite congregation that nurtured their faith.

In many respects my parents were far more open in heart and mind than many of their contemporaries in the church. They were remarkably hospitable. Everyone was welcome at their table regardless of religion, race, economic resources, or social status. Whether friend, neighbor, or transient, all were treated with respect and welcomed into their home.

I returned to Hesston in autumn 1947 for my sophomore year and hoped to continue until graduation in 1950. It was not to be. When it was time for school to begin in autumn 1948, it became apparent that I needed to make the difficult decision to work for the next several years before going back to Hesston.

12

September 1950–June 1956

Attraction, Marriage, and Early Career Goals

Ray and I met at Hesston College in the fall of 1950, when he was a freshman in college and I was a senior in high school. He stopped me one day in the library for a chat. I noticed his eyes, clear and blue as the Kansas sky. His brown wavy hair added to his attraction. Ray Showalter was a handsome young man, a gentleman. He was known for wearing bow ties and dressing impeccably. His clothes were always immaculate with colors perfectly coordinated.

We had our first date on Ray's twenty-first birthday and were soon dating regularly. As I learned to know him, I became aware of something about him that I could not name but thought of as "the wound." I never alluded to it in conversation but assumed that the wound would be healed if I could love him well enough. Was I being naive? Certainly. A little grandiose? Yes, that too. Perhaps most of us believe we can achieve what we perceive as the ideal when we are in love. I was equally aware of my wounds and particularly that I craved love and affection to such a degree that I wasn't sure it could ever be satisfied.

I also discovered that Ray was interested in a career in nursing. He completed his first semester at the college, then transferred to the Kansas City General Hospital School of Nursing in Kansas City, Missouri, in early January. He was going back to the hospital where he had been an orderly three years earlier. We kept our relationship alive by correspondence until Easter, then discontinued our contact for six months.

Another incident that proved to be of critical significance for me in the fall of 1950 was the unexpected, sudden death of my oldest brother. Sam left a wife and six young children. His wife had only an eighth-grade education with no means of earning a living adequate to support her family. Seeing her family break up with several of the children taken into the homes of relatives made me determined to pursue a profession that would make it possible to support a family if I ever needed to.

I completed both my junior and senior years of high school in one year, graduating at age twenty-one in June 1951. Going to college was out of the question because of finances.

I was a member of the college choir that toured for two and a half weeks after graduation. A classmate and I shared a seat one day and talked about future plans as our bus sped through the countryside. She had plans to go to the Mennonite Hospital in La Junta, Colorado, after the tour and study X-ray technology. In an offhand manner, she said, "If I don't like it, I'll let you know and you can take my place." I didn't take the remark seriously, and went home to Ohio for the summer. In August I received a letter from her. She said she was quitting the program; and if I was interested, the director of the program was open to my coming after New Year, 1952.

I arrived in La Junta on January 2 to begin studies in X-ray technology. I lived in the nurse's residence and shared a room with a student laboratory technician. She had also been a student at Hesston but not someone I knew well. We had fun learning to know each other. We took our meals in the hospital dining room.

Ray and I had resumed our letter writing the previous October, and he came to see me in Ohio for the Christmas holidays. Six weeks after I arrived in La Junta, the buzzer in my room sounded one Sunday morning, I was told someone wanted to see me in the lobby. I hurried downstairs. Much to my surprise Ray was waiting for me. He had taken an all-night train from Kansas City to spend the day with me. As we talked he suggested I transfer to the X-ray technology program at Kansas City General, where he was a student nurse. I applied to the program and six weeks later was in Kansas City, Missouri.

Going to Kansas City was my first foray into living and working in a large city. I was fresh from the farm, a novice through and through. I almost shudder remembering how little I knew about life. I knew and understood little enough about my own life, let alone knowing how to relate to the world outside the sheltered communities where I had lived. However, in that *foreign* environment I experienced, for the first time, the grace of acceptance and respect for the person I was rather than having to conform to the expectations of others. It is a gift I have treasured ever since.

I soon learned that my coworkers were real people, that is, the people I worked with knew the pain of loss, disappointments, family problems, and loneliness—the ordinary and not so ordinary difficulties and joys of life. They enjoyed laughter and love and hoped to find meaning in life even as I did. It was a fellow X-ray student, a devout Roman Catholic, who promised to offer her prayers for me as she and I approached the time to write our registry examinations. Her promise created a vital bond between us that nudged me to ask myself, who am I to say that God hears my prayers and not hers? I am ashamed to admit that in my small world we were not accustomed to thinking of Catholics as Christians. But in offering me her prayers, my fellow student had planted a seed of change in my heart—the first among so many seeds planted by others over the years—that slowly enlarged my vision of life, of God, and of God's activity in the world. Today I marvel at the hidden, silent growth that occurs without our awareness, until years later we begin to see the fruit by the changes in our lives.

I have known for years that my love of living in the city is rooted in the positive relationships I enjoyed in the X-ray department of Kansas City General Hospital. My friends there are part of "a great cloud of witnesses" who have contributed to making my life what it has been and is becoming. The work in that place was part of the early preparation for the work I would do years later.

The quiet lawns of a nearby park in the city were the perfect place for a leisurely stroll following a hot day of work inside a hospital with no air conditioning. Ray and I often took long walks in the evening, sometimes taking a break on the front porch swing of good friends before going to our respective homes—single sleeping rooms—close by. It was on that porch swing on a warm July evening after our walk that Ray asked me to marry him. I said yes, and with that yes our world opened into new possibilities. We began to think in terms of we and our instead of I and my.

Ray was halfway through his three-year nursing program when we were engaged, while I had scarcely begun my two years of study. We looked at our schedules and realized that a wedding was in the distant future unless we snatched the one opportunity available in February 1953. We asked for and received the needed approval by the directors of our respective departments. We were pleased with their approval, but we faced one more hurdle as we considered a wedding date. Ray's parents and mine were in Florida for the winter. When we told them we were considering a wedding in February, both couples decided they did not want to return to Kansas City in the middle of the winter even for a wedding. Although we were deeply disappointed, we decided to proceed with our plans.

My brother John agreed to officiate at the wedding and my brother Clarence walked me down the aisle. One of Ray's brothers served as a groomsman and my sister Elizabeth was my matron of honor.

The date for our wedding was set for a Friday evening with the weekend for a short honeymoon. Ray insisted we not see each other on our wedding day until I walked down the aisle. He and three friends completed all the last-minute preparations for the reception. I was relieved of all such duties. Every few hours during the day he called to say, "Remember, we have an appointment at 6:30 this evening." His sister had spent part of the day with him. She told me after his death that on our wedding day he had said to her, "I'm so scared, I'm so scared." She assumed he was having a normal case of the jitters most young people experience before saying, "I do." Perhaps that is all he had in mind; but looking back now, it seems unlikely.

Our honeymoon took us to the Ozark Mountains, where spring flowers were already in bloom. The drive was beautiful. To be away from the city and from the frantic pace of preparing for the wedding was a pleasant relief, yet not everything went according to plan. I was completely taken by surprise when, on the second morning, Ray blocked me when I went to hop into the shower with him. He let me know he would not take a shower or tub bath with me. I felt ashamed, assuming I had been too aggressive.

After the honeymoon, we returned to our work and studies. At the same time, we were eager to start a family and were both delighted when we learned five months after the wedding that I was pregnant. Ray completed his program and passed his State Board of Nursing examinations to become a registered nurse a few months before the birth of our daughter Krista.

I was not allowed to work in the diagnostic X-ray rooms during my pregnancy to prevent possible exposure to radiation. Instead, I worked in the X-ray therapy department, since I was always safely outside the treatment room. I had to return for five months of study and work after Krista was born. I was able to complete the program requirements and write my board examinations in December 1954. The day the letter arrived notifying me that I had passed the exams was a day to celebrate. We had both met our early career goals.

Ray advanced rapidly in his career after receiving his nursing license. He was appointed as head nurse on a thirty-bed surgical ward almost immediately after passing his examinations. He was a highly skilled nurse with exceptional organizational abilities as well. Within a few months he was promoted to assistant director of nursing service.

The graduation exercise for the school of nursing was in May. Ray graduated with highest honors, both academically and clinically. Our three-month-old daughter and I were the only family members present. Ray was disappointed that none of his family came to the ceremony. Several years later, he noticed his father still carried in his billfold a clipping from the hometown newspaper that reported Ray's graduation honors. But never a word passed between them recognizing his success.

Ray thrived on new challenges and did not rest on his laurels. He took evening classes at a nearby college to work toward a bachelor's degree. In addition he regularly scanned professional journals for interesting job possibilities. A particular ad caught his attention, and he submitted his résumé. Following the interview process, he was offered and accepted the position of assistant director of nursing service at Akron Children's Hospital in Akron, Ohio. We were expecting our second child when Ray began the interview process. In early June the following year we were on our way to Ohio with our three-month-old baby Karen and two-year-old Krista.

13

June 1956–June 1966

Ten Years of Transition

We stayed in Ohio for only nine months before packing up and moving to Puerto Rico under the auspices of our denominational mission agency. Ray was called to be director of nursing in the Mennonite hospital in Aibonito.

We stepped off the prop plane into the hot, humid air of San Juan, the capital of Puerto Rico. The sights, sounds, and smells reminded us quickly that we were foreigners. My sister Tillie and her husband met us at the airport. They were completing a five-year term as houseparents in a boys' home with another service agency. Their cement house with tile floors and little lizards running up the walls was another reminder we were no longer in Ohio.

After six weeks of language study for four hours daily, Ray started his work in the hospital and I cared for our two daughters. I soon discovered that memorizing verb conjugations from file cards and ironing little girl's dresses went well together. We were happy to see how quickly our two little girls learned Spanish as they played with the neighbor girls. They also seemed to enjoy being out of doors year round.

Living and working in a crosscultural setting, striving to learn Spanish, and getting to know and understand the people in their cultural context was both enlightening and challenging. The Puerto Rican people are friendly and hospitable. We became especially aware of the generosity of the poor. A poor widow donated her only rooster to be auctioned off to raise money for the churches. A farmer who was a friend of ours sent his son to bring us corn from his garden even though he had eight children to support. The trip between his home and ours was a three-hour journey each way by public bus.

During our second year in Puerto Rico, we offered to provide foster care for a three-month-old baby girl who needed special care because of allergies and severe diarrhea. With her smiles, her silky black curls, and her deep brown eyes, she soon wrapped herself around our hearts. When her parents decided they were not able to provide the special care she needed, it was easy to choose to make her a permanent part of our family. Thus, Carmen became our third daughter. Since I had grown up with four brothers, I wanted a boy to complete our family of four children. A few months before Carmen was two, we had the opportunity to receive a newborn baby boy we named Thomas Ray.

During our fourth year in Aibonito, Ray began to talk about the possibility of returning to the United States. He felt it necessary to return stateside to further his education. Although a desire to go to college lay dormant within me, I could not fully appreciate Ray's commitment to education.

This decision to leave the island was difficult for me. I loved Puerto Rico and had envisioned a long time of mission service there. My family of origin did not see higher education as a priority but had high regard for mission work. For me our call to Puerto Rico was the answer to an inner call to mission service I had received ten years earlier while I was a student at Hesston. I'm not sure I had ever told Ray about that earlier call. I often found it difficult to talk with Ray about things that were especially close to my heart. I never knew if he would say anything in response or be silent. Silence was what I feared most.

We moved from Puerto Rico to North Newton, Kansas, where Ray enrolled in summer school at Bethel College as the first step toward completing his bachelor's degree the following spring.

Our children were one, three, five, and seven when we moved to North Newton. Krista was ready for second grade and Karen would be in kindergarten. We rented a partly furnished two-bedroom apartment, one half of a duplex. Fortunately we did not know in advance how difficult that year would become.

In the middle of July after arriving in North Newton, I was diagnosed with viral pneumonia and admitted to a hospital in Wichita on complete bed rest for two weeks. I was physically and emotionally exhausted. I spent a total of eight weeks in the hospital that year and had to depend on friends, family, and eventually on hired help to care for our children and the house.

In the course of my illness, I was introduced to psychotherapy for the first time. I took the first steps toward opening my pain to another human being. The steps were tentative, to be sure, but a beginning. In one of my last conversations with the psychiatrist, he suggested that Ray was probably latently homosexual (earlier he had met with both of us several times), meaning that his sexual interests and impulses were toward men, even if he was not actively pursuing those interests. I froze inside. I do not recall if I made any verbal response. This possibility was too overwhelming to contemplate. As much as possible I avoided thinking about it, which means I did think about it, with no idea of the implications for our marriage.

The *positive* outcome for me following that wrenching year was that I realized I could choose to pay attention to my emotional health or become ill over and over in the future. I made the decision to pay attention to my emotional needs. My illness and decision to choose life kept me on high alert for resources, whether written or interpersonal, that would help me move toward greater health. Initially, my progress was slow, but I have never regretted the decision.

Ray graduated from Bethel College in early June 1962. He had applied for and received a grant to pursue a master's degree at the University of Oregon in Portland.

Three days after Ray's graduation we went to court in the morning to complete the adoption proceedings for Carmen and Tom, and in the afternoon we left for Portland. It was a long two thousand miles with three adults—a niece of mine went to Oregon with us—four children and a dog in a robin-egg-blue Ford Falcon.

We spent our first night in Oregon with friends living in Corvallis. They cared for the children on Saturday while Ray and I drove to Portland to locate housing. We found a nice house on "hospital hill," close to the university, where Ray reported for his classes on Monday morning as scheduled.

When we arrived in Portland, I drew a deep breath and said to myself, "Home at last!" I was ready to stay put for a loooong time. We had been wanderers for too many years. I wanted roots, not the kind that sprout quickly in thin soil and then wither as quickly. I wanted roots like those of giant trees that sink their roots deep into the earth for the nutrients needed to develop a root system strong enough to withstand the worst of storms. I did not yet understand that it is the *storms* of life that can cause us to reach deeper for the true Source of strength, courage, and hope.

With Ray in graduate school we needed extra income. My niece, who lived with us, preferred taking care of Tom and Carmen, our preschool children, rather than working outside the home. I decided to look for a position in X-ray. Five years had passed since I had worked as a technician, and I had lost a great deal of self-confidence, not only professionally but in many areas of my life. The owner of a twenty-seven-bed private hospital interviewed me and offered the position on the spot.

It turned out to be exactly the therapy I needed. I was the only technician, working with a radiologist five mornings a week for the routine diagnostic procedures. Even during my first week he expressed appreciation for the quality of my work. I scarcely knew how to respond since I had received so little positive feedback for anything I had done in the previous five years. My confidence grew little by little as my skill level improved day by day.

Ray had completed the theoretical requirements for his degree at the end of the first year and accepted a teaching position at the university. He taught full time, did his research, and wrote his thesis during the second year, graduating in spring 1964 with a master's degree in nursing education and administration.

Following graduation he continued teaching at the university and worked three evening shifts a week in a hospital in Portland. I was aware that he was repeating a pattern of overwork I had observed during our four years in Puerto Rico. In both settings we had precious little time together as a family.

Church had always been important to us. We soon located a Mennonite church in Portland. The congregation was in transition, awaiting new pastoral leadership. The new pastor and his family arrived about one year after we did. Our introduction to Marcus and Dottie occurred on the first Sunday after their arrival. Marcus preached that day, and for the first time Jesus became a flesh-and-blood human being for me. His message has stayed with me all these years. The manner in which he prayed is equally memorable. Marcus prayed as if speaking to an intimate friend, which is, of course, what he was doing. No pretense, or special prayer voice, or words to impress, just heart to heart, honest speech. I took careful notice and waited for more.

The "more" I waited and listened for from Marcus came in a later sermon on communication. He said, "It is a sin not to communicate." I wanted to say, "Stop right there. I need to talk about that." His words struck a painful chord in my soul. Since it isn't proper to interrupt a preacher in midsentence, I wrote the quote on a scrap of paper and added, "I don't know if I buy this." It was simple to release the note into his hand when we shook hands as we were leaving the sanctuary. Nothing happened. I got no response. By the latter part of the week, I could wait no longer. I called and set a date for him and his wife to make a home visit. I felt alone and overwhelmed with the responsibility for our family, with little support from Ray because of his heavy work schedule. The afternoon Marcus and Dottie arrived, the three of us sat around the dining room table. For the first time ever, I spilled out years of pent-up hurt, disappointment, loneliness, confusion, and anger, although I could not have named the anger.

When all the venting was over, Marcus did not analyze or interpret but asked a question. "Ann, do you have faith that God can change any of this?"

I heard myself say, "No, I don't." My abdominal muscles contracted as the image of a wagging finger pointed at me saying, "Ann, you should *never* doubt God. God can do *anything*."

Marcus continued, "Ann, God doesn't expect you to have that kind of faith. That is what the church community is for, to have faith for us when we are unable to have faith for ourselves."

The notion that other members in the church could have faith for us when we can no longer believe for ourselves was completely foreign to me. The surprise, relief, and grace of his words were a healing balm. They communicated more than I could assimilate at the moment. That kind of acceptance and grace was new. The words of Marcus and what he modeled became life-changing. He planted seeds of self-acceptance, and his ongoing ministry set me on a journey of self-discovery and self-disclosure that pointed me in a new direction.

My primary image of God had always been that of a stern judge. That image was slowly transformed into one of a loving, compassionate God who is present with us whether we recognize faith within or are without faith at a given time.

Marcus and Dottie also taught me something new about the church as a caring community. Marcus asked, on that unforgettable day, what I thought might happen if Dottie and I met weekly to visit and pray together. I could not imagine anything more helpful. I grabbed for the possibility as a drowning person grabs for a life preserver. His suggestion made concrete his words concerning the role of the church in our lives. Dottie was present for the whole conversation and we agreed then and there to meet regularly. Our getting together each week did not change my circumstances, but the support we gave each other brought renewed faith and courage.

Concern for Carmen prompted me to seek help at child-guidance clinic. My concern for her was sincere, but I also hoped to find help for Ray and me. After a thorough assessment of Carmen, the focus shifted from her to the stress between the two of us. The therapist suggested we begin therapy to relieve stress and improve communication between us. Our progress was slow. Ray went to the sessions but participated only minimally in the conversations. After six months, the therapist told us we were not receiving our money's worth, not during the therapy session or at home between sessions, since we rarely engaged in substantive conversations.

During the two weeks between appointments, I was determined to initiate significant conversation with Ray. I reminded him of the therapist's observation. I can still see him lower his head on the dining room table as he said, "I know I have a strong homosexual orientation, but I have never been untrue to you." I had no reason to doubt either statement. I responded with a lame comment that was not helpful.

Had we managed to engage in a significant conversation? Ray had certainly offered notable information, but neither of us knew the next sentence. I still had no idea what this might mean for our relationship, and I did not know how or what kind of questions to ask to help us explore the implications for our marriage. I was fearful and lacked the skills to take the conversation further.

During our next session with the therapist, I asked Ray to tell him what he had told me and he did. "If that is the case," the therapist responded, "that will be the underlying issue no matter what else we might be discussing." I assumed this would become part of our future conversations. It never did. I was not courageous enough to bring up the subject again, and Ray certainly was not ready to talk further about it. We discontinued therapy as a couple several months later when Ray left Oregon for Kansas. Thus the topic was never raised again for the *eigh teen years* that elapsed between the conversation with the therapist and the day Ray said, "I have AIDS."

What prevented me from raising the issue later? When something is too fearful to examine, it is easy to resort to fantasy—maybe it is no longer true. Maybe he can change if only he tries harder. Or maybe if I can just be better, nicer, kinder, or more attractive, he will be interested in me. Furthermore, no one I knew was discussing homosexuality in the mid-1960s. Without the support of our therapist, I was unable to examine the impact of Ray's sexual orientation on our marriage. (Years later I realized a therapist cannot force a couple to discuss a topic they are unwilling or unable to discuss.) To do so would have been like looking directly at the sun at high noon—blinding.

I was both ignorant and unable to accept something considered as shameful and humiliating as homosexuality. I know of nothing that raises more hostility, fear, disgust, disrespect, and rejection in the general public than same-sex orientation and behavior.

The powerful messages from my past—that if there are problems of a sexual nature in a marriage, the wife is at fault—contributed to the long silence. However, the most significant factor was the degree to which my identity as a woman had been undermined. I found it almost impossible to feel that I was desirable as a person after being pushed away innumerable times when I wanted to offer Ray a hug or a kiss.

Through indescribable pain and disappointments beyond telling, I had learned that Ray's first defense against discussing anything uncomfortable was silence. That was true of matters far less personal or threatening than same-sex orientation. Consequently, in the last few years of our marriage, I always had to consider whether or not I could tolerate silence as a response before raising anything of consequence to me.

The president of Hesston College had begun a conversation with Ray during our third year in Oregon, urging him to consider a position on the college faculty. He wanted Ray, along with colleagues, to design a two-year program in nursing education that would prepare students to write the state board examinations to become registered nurses. If students passed the exams, they were ready for the job market in two years. Ray was energized by the new challenge. I knew from the beginning he was intrigued by and wanted the position. He had the credentials and experience needed to give direction to such a program. Again I was the one to hold back. I could not bear to think of leaving Oregon. After holding out for a year, I agreed to another move but with great internal resistance.

Moving to Kansas was going home for Ray and had the added appeal of establishing a new program at the college and teaching in the place where both of us had been students. Furthermore, it reinforced his commitment to the church and its institutions. I also wonder if it could have been another attempt to hold the family together and maintain the appearance that everything was normal. I raise the possibility not as an indictment against Ray but as a search to understand more fully the dynamics of our relationship.

Ray left for Hesston in March 1966 because he needed to be on the campus for six months before accepting the first students, which the college wanted to do in September. He and his colleagues designed a program they believed would serve both the college and the community. The years since then have proved many times over that their knowledge and instincts were correct.

In order for the children to finish the school year, I stayed with them in Oregon. Ray and I had agreed I would continue seeing the therapist because I needed the support while being alone with the children and preparing for the move. The three months until June flew by quickly. We needed to sell our house and were fortunate to know of friends returning from a term of service in Africa at almost the same time we would be moving. They bought the house sight unseen, with all negotiations accomplished by mail. I packed our belongings and made arrangements for a rental truck. Several young men from our church drove the truck to Kansas for us. We said our good-byes in early June to start the long trek to south-central Kansas.

I was in mourning as I clung to the last glimpse of majestic Mount Hood. I felt hollow inside. We unloaded our belongings in Hesston ten years after beginning the journey from Kansas City, Missouri, to Ohio. A long period of self-pity followed.

Lord,
it isn't easy
to speak the truth
in love. It's much easier
to hide from one another and
call that love. But I confess today
that that is not love, but fear which breeds
distrust and suspicion. At the same time I admit
how easy it is to become self-righteous and how hard
it is to see things from another's point of view. I
pray that today each of us may, in a new way,
listen to each other and with new openness
believe that you can make yourself known
among us through both confrontation
and acceptance, through both
judgment and grace.

14

July 1966–August 1978

Heartaches and Arrangements

During my senior year in seminary in 1982, I was in a seminar group. The group had experienced a time of painful conflict when it was my turn to prepare the opening worship and lead in prayer. I had written the prayer on the back of a used envelope with no thought that anyone would be particularly interested in it. After the seminar one of my classmates asked for a copy of the prayer. I handed him the envelope. On commencement day he brought me an elegant page of parchment with the prayer transcribed in calligraphy. Ray had it framed for me and it hangs on the wall next to my computer and now is on the facing page of this chapter. It seemed an appropriate prayer to place at the beginning of "Heartaches and Arrangements."

As always, Ray invested himself wholeheartedly in his work. He taught nursing courses as well as giving oversight to the program. He was determined to maintain close ties with the president, the dean, and other faculty members involved in designing the program. Their continued support and counsel was crucial to the long-term development and success of the program.

My sense of being rootless returned. I was bereft of a trusted pastor and his wife, who was a good friend and companion with me on the spiritual journey. I felt understood and challenged by the therapist and trusted him. The internal image of my life at the time was that I had been climbing a long, steep hill on a narrow, winding path. I was nearing the crest when it was time to move, and I was afraid of sliding all the way back to the starting place. The losses were real, not just imagined, and little by little I discovered the gains were real as well. I did not slide back to the starting point.

Several months after arriving in Hesston, I wrote a long letter to my former therapist complaining about all my losses and Ray's inadequacies. He took his time in responding, but he did respond. First, he put his finger on my self-pity to help me see it was not serving me well. He pointed out that Ray was responsible for anything he said or did that was not kind, gentle, understanding, or truthful, and I was responsible for how it affected me. I'm not sure a fist in the stomach could have hurt more. It was not what I expected, but I mulled it over because I trusted his intention and knowledge. After weeks of ruminating, I realized he meant to tell me I was not a victim. I was free to choose my responses, thus creating a new reality. His were words of great wisdom.

Understanding that message was a beginning point but not the destination. Old patterns of response were difficult to overcome, but persistent practice over time began to make a difference. It was like learning a difficult piece of music. Consistent practice creates beautiful music, even if the tempo or the dynamics are not quite perfect or not exactly like another person's interpretation of the score.

Two ventures during our first year in Hesston helped me adjust to our new environment. I went to the local mental health center and participated in group therapy. The feedback of other group members added a new ingredient to therapy that brought helpful insights. It was equally useful to join the conversation as others worked on their problems. Furthermore, finding help through the local facility reassured me there were resources available to help with climbing the hills that lay ahead.

The second venture fulfilled a dream that had been hidden away in my heart since junior high school. Unknown to family and friends, I had a yen to participate in drama, something that was never possible for a young Amish girl.

Hesston was home to a large farm machinery manufacturing company. The wife of the president of the company announced plans for a community theater production. The play she chose was a spoof on big business. When she invited people to audition, I went and was given the leading role. I'm not sure anyone else auditioned for the part. It mattered not a whit. To imagine myself in the character of another and allow myself to speak through the voice of a woman whose assertiveness I admired was therapeutic far beyond my expectations when I decided to audition. The discipline and teamwork required to hone the production was rewarding in itself, but the biggest thrill of all was to participate in three well-done performances. Allowing myself to enjoy the applause was frosting on the cake. But my yen was not satisfied by a single drama. For the next six years, I participated in theater each year. I had found a new voice.

Ray's organizational skills and commitment to giving his best made him a gifted administrator. He was friendly and outgoing, possessed a sharp intellect, was observant of his surroundings and possessed a memory for detail that was extraordinary. He met strangers easily and rarely forgot a face or a name.

However, when carried to extremes, our best gifts often become liabilities. Ray was a perfectionist and a workaholic, a slave to detail. His perfectionism demanded that he work hours and hours beyond what any employer demanded. Most of his adult life he worked several jobs at once.

Ray wanted to build a new house after living in a rental for a year. From past experience of living in a house while doing major renovation, I imagined us painting the walls and doing all the finish work on the kitchen cabinets after moving in. I was not keen on undertaking a building project. However, Ray promised that everything would be completed before we moved into the new house. That was what I needed to hear. We went to the building site together every day but two from the day the builder dug the first hole until the completion of the project. It turned out to be an enjoyable venture.

We had a comfortable new house, yet Ray did not succeed in finding a home in himself. During his fourth year at the college he came home from work one day and announced he was planning to work toward a second masters degree, this one in medical anthropology. The University of Kansas in Lawrence had substantial grants available for nurses working on advanced degrees. Relying on the grant monies made it financially feasible for him to further his education. However, it also meant he would be away from home every week Monday through Friday for the entire school year.

He continued as director of the nursing department at the college while pursuing his courses at the university. His weekends at home were consumed with his work in the nursing department, except for Sunday morning, which he reserved to attend church with the family. He had completed the academic requirements for the degree by the end of the following summer but never completed a thesis.

At that point Ray resigned his position at the college to accept a new appointment as educational consultant for the Kansas State Board of Nursing in Topeka. With our two older children in high school and another in special education, it was not a suitable time to move the family again. Ray commuted to his work in Topeka for seven years, coming home only on weekends. I took him to meet the train at 10:30 Sunday nights, then met the 4:30 train on Friday mornings to pick him up. In addition he worked two evenings each weekend at a local hospital.

Ray's decision to resign his position at the college to work in Topeka precipitated a crisis for me. I thought of our relationship as suffering from an internal cancer. The crisis sent me into two years of therapy. Gradually the focus in therapy shifted from Ray to my own issues, and slowly I learned to take more responsibility for my feelings and actions.

Despite the pain, my prayers, my work in therapy, and my special friends kept a flicker of hope alive. Like the prophet Isaiah's "dimly burning wick" (42:3), that flicker of hope was never completely extinguished. Was the process painful? Absolutely. Did I ever wonder if God was hearing my prayers? Indeed I did. Often I wondered how to cope day by day. Frequently I felt sorry for myself. Yet God's love remained constant, giving me strength to do what I needed to.

The years in Hesston were midlife years. Weathering the challenges of guiding our four children through the ups and downs of elementary school, adolescence, and high school, alone most of the time, was an arduous responsibility. I experienced the midlife chaos in fear and trembling, as Krista approached high school graduation. The unanswered question was, what will I do when the children are gone? I hadn't a clue.

I chose to try a variety of tasks in the church during those years. I sang in the choir, served as secretary of the women's group, directed children's choir for a year, served on church council, taught high school youth in Sunday school, and served as director of adult Christian education. In the process I discovered tasks that fit my interests and skills, those I enjoyed doing and those I didn't care to repeat. So I invested my energies in the activities that fit and said no to those that did not.

My pastor, Jerry Weaver, encouraged me in many ways, even suggesting in one conversation that perhaps some day I would go to seminary. The idea was so far removed from the reality of my life that for twenty years I forgot the conversation had taken place. It was only when Jerry and I worked together in 1993 as pastors of First Mennonite Church in Denver, Colorado, that I remembered the conversation from the early 1970s.

I also experimented with a variety of jobs during those years. X-ray technology was too mechanical for me to make it a lifelong career. The acting dean at Hesston College called one day and invited me to be his secretary. That led to serving as administrative assistant in the general education department at the college.

There was no way for me to know during those chaotic, excruciating midlife years that all my exploration of interests and skills, the variety of work in the church and at the college, was of much greater worth than anything I could have dreamed in a lifetime. Nothing was wasted. Instead something new, surprising, and life-giving was being created ready to unfold in "the fullness of time." The first part of the surprise was about to be unveiled.

15

My College and Career

My desire to go to college had been silent—most of the time—as if asleep, waiting for the right time to waken. The summer of our tenth anniversary in Hesston, Ray and I decided the time had come for me to stop working outside the home and enroll in a few college courses for personal enrichment. Working toward a degree was not in our thoughts at all.

Through the registrar at Hesston College, I learned that Bethel College, in nearby North Newton, had a special program for adults whereby they assigned college credit for work experience if the person was able to demonstrate competencies in the various areas of general education. I made an appointment to meet with the director of the program. He explained the kinds of materials required for evaluation. I spent three weeks assembling the materials and submitted them. After evaluating the materials, the director of the program granted sixty-six hours of credit to be validated by work in the classroom. That meant I could complete the requirements for a bachelor's degree in two years. I was ecstatic.

I decided to pursue a degree in social work, hoping later to complete a master's degree in clinical social work to become a therapist. Jerry Weaver, my former pastor in Hesston, had become campus pastor at Bethel College. He saw me during registration and suggested I consider going to our denominational seminary in Elkhart, Indiana, for an introductory course in ministry during the January interterm. Going to Elkhart for three weeks seemed impossible, yet the course would fulfill the requirement for an upper-level Bible course.

Ultimately Ray arranged to be at home during those three weeks, making it possible for me to go to Elkhart. The assignment for our final day of the course was to come prepared to share our professional direction with a small seminar group.

"I plan to complete a master's degree in clinical social work to become a therapist," I said when it was my turn. Several men in the class who had undergraduate degrees in social work questioned the wisdom of the direction I was planning.

"Are you sure that's what you should be doing?" one of them asked.

Shrugging, I said, "I think so. I don't know what else."

"I've seen gifts in you during these three weeks that will not be used in social work," said another.

The professor turned to me and asked, "Ann, have you ever considered pastoral ministry?"

I couldn't believe what I was hearing. At the time I knew of only one ordained woman in the branch of the Mennonite church I belonged to.

"Well, no," I burst out, then stopped. My next response was far more subdued: "I've known for many years that, had I been a man, I would have been a pastor." It was the first time the intuitive knowing had been voiced.

"Isn't it interesting," said the professor, "that when the gifts for ministry are present in your brothers (I had two brothers who were ministers) they can be recognized; but when the gifts are present in you, they can't be."

Something profound awoke in me in that brief interchange, but I had no idea what it meant. Two days later I returned home and said nothing about the conversation to anyone, including Ray. In effect I put the comments into a cubbyhole and said, "Lord, I have no idea what this means or what to do with it." Then I went off to my classes at Bethel and waited.

Within the next eight months two other people spoke to me about considering pastoral ministry, perhaps becoming a hospital chaplain. Much to my surprise, when I discussed the idea with Ray, he encouraged me to explore it. One of the friends who had suggested pastoral ministry urged me to speak with the director of pastoral care at the local mental health center. She knew he sometimes accepted a person into the summer chaplaincy program before he or she had attended seminary. I called for an appointment and visited with the director. He was willing to consider my application for the summer program, and I was accepted.

Two weeks after graduating from Bethel College, I began my work in Clinical Pastoral Education (CPE) at Prairie View Mental Health Center in Newton. The work felt as though I had put on a garment that fit perfectly. The ten weeks were over much too quickly. It was time for my final evaluation session with the director. "What do I do now?" I asked.

"If you are serious about becoming a chaplain, you must go to seminary," he answered calmly.

"Please, can't I stay for full year?" I begged.

The director was adamant. "You have to complete at least one year of seminary before I would consider taking you back."

I was disappointed but not despondent. I was grateful for a formative summer. Nothing could take that from me.

Krista and Karen were both married, Carmen was in voluntary service, and Tom was living with friends of the family the summer I completed my work at Prairie View. That meant the nest at home was empty. It was time for me to move to Topeka to be with Ray. The decision was not easy. Our first grandchild was three months old. I went to see her every day since her parents lived nearby. She seemed like such a miracle. Life had come full circle. The life Ray and I had created together had now given life to a new generation. But it wasn't only leaving my daughter's family that gave me pause. I had carved out a niche in the community that was varied and rewarding.

On the other hand, Ray and I had not lived together full time for eight long years. I had to face the honest reservations about what life would be like living together again. Ray was often severely depressed when he came home for a weekend. I wasn't sure I could endure his depression day after day and told him so. I asked that we not sell our house in Hesston but rent it for a year. We could decide then whether or not to sell. We rented the house easily but retained access to a basement bedroom for our use when we returned to Hesston for a visit.

We moved most of our belongings into a two-bedroom apartment in Topeka. It was cozy, convenient, and comfortable with easy access to the downtown area where Ray worked. I began looking for a social work position. Surely someone was waiting with just the right position for me, fresh out of college. Think again, Ann. There were desk jobs available, if I wanted to work with paper most of the time. Not me. I wanted to work with people, not paper. Eventually I took a position as receptionist in the office of two dermatologists. It wasn't what I expected but more interesting than spending most of the day filling out forms.

We enjoyed living in Topeka, found a church where we felt at home, and had several good friends. Over the Christmas and New Year holidays that year Ray complained of not feeling well. His digestive system wasn't up to par, and he felt more tired than usual. Over lunch a few days later, he asked if his eyes looked unusual. When I looked carefully, I saw that his eyes were jaundiced. He called his doctor in Newton and was admitted to the hospital. Hepatitis B. I didn't know how serious the disease was or that it can be sexually transmitted. He was hospitalized for a week, then ordered to stay at home for six weeks. I became the courier between his office and home so that he could carry on his most urgent work. His energy was minimal for months after he went back to the office.

Ray was active in national nursing organizations, a member of the committee that screened and selected the test items for the national registry examination for nurses. When the responsibilities of that committee were to be transferred to a new organization with offices in Chicago in late 1979, the executive director invited Ray to accept a position as associate director. He later was named director of testing and chairperson of the examination committee. He was excited about the new possibility. He had reached the top of his profession and was known nationally for his expertise in nursing education and administration.

I went with Ray to a nursing convention in San Antonio, Texas, in summer 1979. We took a few days to relax and visit places of interest before the convention. It was a delightful several days. We had lunch with the colleague who wanted him to join her staff in Chicago. Who was dragging her feet about another move less than eighteen months after moving to Topeka? Yours truly. Although I enjoyed city living, I thought of Chicago as the last place on earth I wanted to live. The prospect felt intimidating.

Ray's work in Topeka became more and more demanding. We had as little time together as ever, and he saw no hope for relief in the future. Work took precedence over everything else. A journal entry speaks to the issue.

> Ray is involved with another woman. Her name is Work. I've met her before but had almost forgotten her during our time away. We spent such good time together. I was content and happy with him. I hoped he would find enough joy in our companionship that he would treat Work as secondary. It was not to be. He is once again consumed by her charms. She apparently offers him a sense of self worth, and a position of honor and prestige among his colleagues. In addition she pays

him a handsome salary. It's very strange she allows him to freely share his money with me. No sign of jealousy!

I knew he was working too hard but wondered how a new position in Chicago with greater responsibility could be less demanding. We also had decided that I would begin seminary studies in Kansas City, Kansas, in September. It was a sixty-mile commute, but housing at reasonable cost was available on campus where commuters could spend several nights a week. I was eager to get started, but the thought of transferring to a seminary in the Chicago area in the middle of the first year was distressing.

Once Ray had made the decision to accept the position in Chicago, it made sense to move between Christmas and New Year. I had made arrangements to transfer to Bethany Theological Seminary in Oak Brook, a Chicago suburb. Student housing was available on campus, greatly simplifying our move. We could get acquainted with the city and take our time deciding where to settle more permanently.

Ray drove our car, and a son-in-law drove the truck with our belongings. I delayed my departure for a week as daughter Carmen had delivered a new baby several weeks earlier, and I wanted to spend the extra week with her before taking the train to the windy city.

Entering the city of Chicago on the train can be depressing; the route took me through a major industrial section of the city before reaching Union Station. The late afternoon sky was cloudy and gray. A layer of black grime covered the snow, leaving it as gray as the clouds overhead. I let myself feel as ugly and uninviting as the landscape. I did not want to move to Chicago, and this view of the city confirmed my distaste. A strange thing occurred as I wallowed in my dark thoughts and impressions. Gradually, at the very edge of perception, I felt my spirit lifting. The resentment I felt about moving to this city slowly faded, and I did not understand why. The scenery had not improved, yet the awareness dawned on me that this journey was all right.

I was mercifully oblivious of the fact that the grayness of the late afternoon with its clouds hanging low over the city was like a silent warning of the dark clouds gathering around our marriage.

Ray met me at Union Station, and we drove through the downtown area. Michigan Avenue was aglow with Christmas lights, and the mammoth tree in Daley Plaza dwarfed any Christmas tree I had ever seen. I had Saturday and Sunday to get acquainted with our new surroundings before seminary classes began on Monday morning.

We soon chose to become part of a congregation in Oak Park, still in its birth throes. The first Sunday we attended, there were only ten of us. However, two single women were nurses from Kansas. It was nice to connect with someone from home. Within a few months we decided to make Oak Park our home. In the spring we bought a condominium that was within walking distance of the elevated train that Ray took downtown to his work, and I made the twelve-mile commute to the seminary.

I decided to explore working with the chaplain at one of the hospitals in Oak Park during the summer to fulfill a field education requirement. Chaplain Bob agreed to work with me for the summer. He nurtured in me a developing pastoral identity, encouraged me to conduct a grief workshop for new nurse assistants, and offered me the opportunity to colead a bereavement support group with him for the following year. I developed friendships with people in the pastoral care department that remained part of my life for many years. Those friendships were especially important since I needed to look outside of our marriage for emotional support and the exchange of ideas. Chaplain Bob and I remain good friends.

Ray showed his support for my seminary work by typing my term papers and typing and assembling the materials I wrote for my comprehensive exams. I experienced more support from him during my years in college and seminary than at any previous time in our marriage. I was licensed for ministry (the first step toward ordination in our denomination) the same day I graduated from seminary. Ray stood at my side as I made my vows.

"In my Father's house there are many dwelling places. If it were not so, would I have told you that I go to prepare a place for you?" (Jesus, in John 14:2). Usually we read this passage as referring to our future life in heaven. Without denying that possibility, I wonder if we do not shortchange ourselves when we fail to consider that Jesus also prepares a place for us here and now. It seems so as I review my life.

On September 1, 1982, I began a one-year residency in Clinical Pastoral Education at Rush-Presbyterian—St. Luke's Medical Center in Chicago. It was a place of preparation, I assumed, for ministry as a hospital chaplain. It became that and so much more. The daily exposure to suffering and death pushed me to examine what it means to be present with people in the most vulnerable situations in life.

Learning that two of our supervising chaplains were gay men—one a Roman Catholic priest and the other a Protestant minister—stretched me to consider who God calls to be his ministering servants. There were times I felt stretched physically, emotionally, and spiritually almost to a breaking point.

Our supervisors suggested early in the year that each of us go into therapy since we were likely to meet in our patients the unfinished issues in our own lives. Problems with authority, sexuality, fear, death, and anger could easily interfere with our ministry if we left them unexamined. I soon discovered the wisdom of their suggestion.

The timid little Amish girl inside of me was terrified of the strange world of a major medical center. She was terrified of the sheer numbers of new faces she saw day after day—doctors, nurses, social workers, and medical residents—many of whom she perceived as authority figures and therefore intimidating. I tried to no avail to hold her fear at bay by an act of the will. She kept me so fearful that it was difficult to go to the pediatric unit to visit sick and dying children and meet parents devastated by grief, disappointment, anxiety, and anger.

Father Jim Corrigan was the supervisor we four residents met with weekly. One day during our supervisory session I knew I had to pay attention to my frightened child. I admitted the depth of my fear to the group. Then I turned in my chair as though facing a person and said: "Annie [the name I gave my frightened child], you no longer need to hide behind your mother's skirt. You don't need to be afraid; you are welcome to go with me to the unit. I'll take care of you." What followed was not a magical healing of all my fears, but I felt a significant change in the level of fear and greater confidence as I went about my work.

A short time later a dear friend sent me a poster she had made of a barefoot girl outdoors in a bandanna, looking with fascination and joy at a rainbow. I put that poster above my desk in my office. The bandanna girl became the symbol of the freedom and joy I wanted for Annie. For the next few years I tried to nurture my inner child, though I no longer remember the specifics of the process. Today Annie is alive and as joyful as the barefoot bandanna girl was. She is the spontaneous, fun-loving part of me, occupying the center of my being where the Spirit is at home.

My work in therapy produced new possibilities and new anxieties. I spent a great deal of energy working through grief related to my childhood. I also invested enormous energy searching how to unlock the mystery that separated Ray and me and prevented the closeness I yearned for. Perhaps the key was to accept with grace what we had in common since we were in a marriage that dared not fail because of faith commitments. Ray and I engaged in less and less meaningful conversation and in less and less emotional and physical intimacy during that year.

The following excerpt from my journal reflects the level of self-doubt I had:

Do I matter? Is it all right that I exist? Do I count anywhere, for anything, for anyone? My head says, yes, my heart and emotions are not sure. There is nothing at the deepest level that says, Ann I'm so glad you exist, you are infinitely significant to me. The problem is not Ray, it's me!

Taking responsibility for "the problem" was a way of maintaining a flicker of hope. Because I knew I could not change Ray, I had to believe there was something I could change in myself to become more acceptable to him. Taking responsibility for the problem also reflects my long denial that Ray's choices and behaviors severely limited our life together. We were caught in a marriage that dared not fail.

The flicker of hope and my efforts to become more acceptable to Ray were doomed to failure, since they did not admit the real problem. However, the day Ray said, "I have AIDS and in recent years have lived as a gay man," all the missing pieces in the puzzle of our life together fell into place. That seed of truth fell into receptive and fertile ground at the core of my being. Recognizing and accepting his truth gave birth to recognizing and owning myself with a certainty that was new.

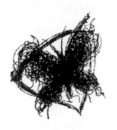

Part Three

How long, O LORD? Will you forget me forever?
How long will you hide your face from me?
How long must I bear pain in my soul,
and have sorrow in my heart all day long?
—Psalm 13:1-2

16

August 1984

Farewell Rituals

The first of the farewell rituals began in the therapist's office when he challenged me to describe the kind of service I would plan if Ray were to die. I did not think of it as a farewell ritual at the time but know now it was just that. Five days after his diagnosis, Ray and I joined in another ritual of farewell as we planned his funeral and memorial services. Krista, Karen, and I added another ritual when we made arrangements with the funeral director and chose the casket. Still later we were engaged in a soulful, eloquent farewell as my chaplain friend sang for us. We were beginning our grieving. Some weeks before Ray's death I contacted the ministers in Kansas we had chosen to lead the private funeral and public memorial service.

I had also asked Jerry Weaver, our former pastor, to include an announcement during the memorial service that Ray had died of AIDS. I was not willing to live with yet another secret—Ray's diagnosis. The Mennonite Church is small compared to mainline denominations in the United States. We had lived in many places: from Ohio to Puerto Rico and from Portland, Oregon, to Chicago and a number of points between. We knew people from across the country, and I was certain I would be asked repeatedly the cause of Ray's death. I was not inclined to make excuses when that happened. Ray and the children had agreed it would be best to make a public announcement. I had also told Ray's family that the announcement would be made so they would not be taken by surprise. The only problem we faced was to know how to do it with dignity and good taste.

We had been members of Whitestone Mennonite Church in Hesston for the twelve years we lived in Hesston from the mid-1960s to the late 1970s. Ray wanted us to close the memorial service with the church choir singing the "Hallelujah Chorus" from Handel's *Messiah*. I had asked Jerry to see if that could be arranged, since the choir did not practice or sing regularly during the summer months. The remaining details for the services were to be arranged when I arrived in Kansas. Every one of those activities helped prepare us for the final rituals after Ray's death. Not only that, planning ahead of time for the final farewell kept us connected with the reality of his approaching death rather than avoiding it.

On Monday, the day after Ray died, Karen and I flew from Chicago to Kansas City, where she had parked her car at the airport. We drove the remaining two hundred miles to Hesston, arriving in time for dinner. When we reached Ray's brother's home, they told me that Jerry and my dear pastor friend Dotty Janzen were waiting for me at the church, ready to plan the services.

The private funeral service, including only our immediate family, our siblings, and a few very close friends, took place on Wednesday morning. The burial was at a small country cemetery twenty-five miles northwest of Hesston, the place where his parents, grandparents, and a host of relatives were buried.

A year earlier, Ray and I and one of his brothers and sister-in-law had visited the cemetery. The two brothers walked past every marker, recalling memories of almost everyone. How ironic that his burial was his homecoming. He had come home to be laid to rest in the company of his extended family, those to whom he could never reveal the person he knew himself to be. Following the burial we returned to the church for a luncheon prepared by the women of the church.

The sanctuary was filled to capacity for the evening memorial service. Early in the service Jerry said that Ray had not been feeling well for many months and that after he was admitted to the hospital for complete medical examinations, Ray's diagnosis was AIDS. Jerry also spoke of the wonderful support our Oak Park congregation had provided during the last few days of Ray's life and the peaceful closure Ray and I had experienced before his death. His few words were appropriate and spoken with dignity and provided all the information necessary.

Six of Ray's professional colleagues from both state and national nursing organizations were present. Several of them paid tribute to Ray's contribution to the nursing profession. The governor of Kansas had sent a letter of condolence in recognition and appreciation for Ray's work as a state employee.

The Scriptures, prayers, and music were uplifting. I had chosen a medley of Scripture passages from the Psalms and the book of Isaiah, passages that speak of human suffering, sin, and need, alternated with messages of forgiveness, redemption, and hope.

A Medley of Pain and Sorrow, of Comfort and Hope

People: Out of the depths I cry to you, O LORD.
Lord, hear my voice!
Let your ears be attentive
to the voice of my supplications!

Pastor: If you, O LORD, should mark iniquities,
Lord, who could stand?
But there is forgiveness with you,
so that you may be revered. (Ps. 130:1-4)

O Israel, hope in the LORD!
For with the Lord there is steadfast love,
and with him is great power to redeem.
It is he who will redeem Israel
from all its iniquities. (Ps. 130:7-8)

People: O LORD, do not rebuke me in your anger,
or discipline me in your wrath!
For your arrows have sunk into me,
and your hand has come down on me.
There is no soundness in my flesh
because of your indignation;
There is no health in my bones
because of my sin.
For my iniquities have gone over my head;
they weigh like a burden too heavy for me. (Ps. 38:1-4)

Pastor: You who live in the shelter of the Most High,
who abide in the shadow of the Almighty,
will say to the LORD, "My refuge and my fortress;
my God, in whom I trust." (Ps. 91:1-2)
You will not fear the terror of the night,
or the arrow that flies by day,
or the pestilence that stalks in darkness,
or the destruction that wastes at noonday. (Ps. 91:5-6)
For he will command his angels concerning you
to guard you in all your ways.
On their hands they will bear you up,
so that you will not dash your foot against a stone.
  (Ps. 91:11-12)

People: My wounds grow foul and fester
because of my foolishness;
I am utterly bowed down and prostrate;
all day I go around mourning.

For my loins are filled with burning,
and there is no soundness in my flesh.
I am utterly spent and crushed;
I groan because of the tumult of my heart. (Ps. 38:5-8)

Pastor: Bless the LORD, O my soul,
and do not forget all his benefits—
who forgives all your iniquity,
who heals all your diseases,
who redeems your life from the Pit,
who crowns you with steadfast love and mercy,
who satisfies you with good as long as you live
so that your youth is renewed like the eagle's. (Ps. 103:2-5)

People: O LORD, do not rebuke me in your anger,
or discipline me in your wrath.
Be gracious to me, O LORD, for I am languishing;
O LORD, heal me, for my bones are shaking with terror.
My soul also is struck with terror,
while you, O LORD—how long? (Ps. 6:1-3)

Pastor: I waited patiently for the LORD;
he inclined to me and heard my cry.
He drew me up from the desolate pit,
out of the miry bog,
and set my feet upon a rock,
making my steps secure.
He put a new song in my mouth,
a song of praise to our God. (Ps. 40:1-3a)

People: Turn, O LORD, save my life;
deliver me for the sake of your steadfast love.
For in death there is no remembrance of you;
in Sheol who can give you praise?
I am weary with my moaning;

every night I flood my bed with tears;
I drench my couch with my weeping. (Ps. 6:4-6)

Pastor: Do not fear, for I have redeemed you;
I have called you by name, you are mine.
When you pass through the waters, I will be with you;
and through the rivers, they shall not overwhelm you;
when you walk through fire you shall not be burned,
and the flame shall not consume you.
For I am the LORD your God,
the Holy One of Israel, your Savior. (Isa. 43:1b-3a)

People: Incline your ear, O LORD, and answer me,
for I am poor and needy.
Preserve my life, for I am devoted to you;
save your servant who trusts in you.
You are my God; be gracious to me, O Lord,
for to you do I cry all day long. (Ps. 86:1-3)

Pastor: Do not fear, for I am with you,
do not be afraid, for I am your God;
I will strengthen you, I will help you,
I will uphold you with my victorious right hand.

For I, the LORD your God,
hold your right hand;
it is I who say to you, "Do not fear,
I will help you. (Isa. 41:10, 13)

Jerry's meditation was filled with God's love and grace, a welcome word to all of us. His text was from the story of the lost son, the prodigal. One of Jerry's comments has remained with me: "The young man came to the realization that what he had left behind was, in fact, what he was most searching for." Later, a colleague of Ray's during the time he was the executive director of the Kansas State Board of Nursing told me Jerry's message had inspired and challenged her to the point of changing her life in significant ways. At the close of the service, the sanctuary resounded with the "Hallelujah Chorus" sung by the church choir. Although we were in deep grief the whole service was an affirmation of Ray's life and our faith.

The public statement that Ray had died of AIDS broke the cultural and social rules of the community, but I have never regretted the decision. When someone asked the cause of his death, I could look the person in the eyes and tell him or her the truth: no hedging, no excuses, no apologies. Word of Ray's diagnosis and subsequent death spread quickly. The announcement apparently gave permission for others to share secrets they had been living with. People were not long in coming to me. Wherever I have gone in the months and years since his death, person after person has come to tell me or in some cases has written that a husband, father, brother, cousin, uncle, mother—or whoever the relative—is lesbian or gay. This came as a surprise. I had not anticipated such a response, though I understand well the relief that comes in finding someone willing to listen and understand without condemnation.

A family member living in Hesston at the time told me later there had been little if any gossip about Ray's diagnosis. Apparently knowing the truth had left little room or need for gossip.

17

The Comfort of Community

Several close friends provided lodging while I waited for family members to arrive for the services. I spent Monday night with Vernon and his wife Dolores. Vernon and Ray first met in high school years ago. Later Ray, Vernon, and Dolores were students and graduates of the same school of nursing. Still later Vernon went to medical school and specialized in psychiatry. Dolores earned a degree in elementary education and is the mother of five children. Our children often played together while growing up.

Dolores was graciously hospitable, someone with whom I could be myself. The three of us had a long conversation about Ray and the circumstances of his death that evening.

"Vernon, it is clear in retrospect that Ray often alluded to his sexual orientation in veiled ways, and I failed to pick up the signals."

"No doubt it is gracious that you did not pick up the allusions. What would either of you have chosen to do about the situation?"

He was right. Painful as life was at times for both of us, neither of us would have chosen divorce as a better option. Years later, when I visited with Dolores and Vernon, they remembered their last visit with Ray. Both had been aware at the time that it seemed like he wanted to tell them something more about himself but for some reason had been unable to.

Tuesday night I stayed with Wayne and Margie. Our history also went back to high school. The friendship grew and was strengthened during the twelve years we lived in Hesston. The three of us talked for hours about homosexuality and the tragedy of Ray's death. Hesston is a town of about 4,000 in south-central Kansas. Same-sex orientation was not a common topic of conversation in that community. Controversial issues, if acknowledged at all, were discussed privately and discreetly.

I awoke early the next morning, dressed, and sat on the front porch swing to absorb the restful silence. The opportunity to listen to the silence was balm for my wounded soul, so intensely stretched to new limits in the recent past. The morning sun inched its way silently above the horizon, a gloriously golden orb. (In Chicago I was accustomed to seeing miles of buildings instead of the horizon.) A few hens, awake with the early light, scratched in the dirt, hoping to find a few fat grubs for breakfast. The dog wandered out of the barn, stretched, then wagged his tail, assuring me all was well before coming to sniff the stranger on the swing. A young goat cavorted on a pile of rocks.

Before I knew she was nearby, Margie plunked a litter of baby kittens into my lap. Life! All around me the morning pulsated with life, reminding me that death does not have the last word. Life goes on even when death asserts itself, taking from us those we love. My heart, aching from the siege of sickness and death, responded with thanksgiving. Good friends are surely to be counted as one of life's greatest gifts.

The opportunity to visit with many friends following the memorial service was reassuring, for they shared memories and words of appreciation for Ray and his work. Their words warmed my heart. To know others who knew Ray and loved him confirmed my love for him.

Friends from Topeka attending the service invited me to go home with them for the night and offered to take me to the airport the next morning for my flight home to Chicago. Krista and Karen were planning to return to Chicago in time for the memorial service at Oak Park, but it was important to me to go home alone before they came. With Ray's death I knew I would be living alone, and I wanted to be alone when I crossed the threshold of my apartment for the first time. There was no reason to delay facing the new reality that I was now a widow.

A young man from our congregation at Oak Park met my plane at O'Hare International when I arrived in Chicago and took me to my apartment in Oak Park. The apartment was filled with reminders of Ray. The reminders brought me closer to Ray and I felt comforted to be at home—alone.

Friday evening, August 10, we celebrated Ray's life in a memorial service at Oak Park. I felt surrounded by love as many friends and colleagues gathered to remember Ray and offer support for my daughters and me. Together they formed the web of life Ray and I had been part of during his life. Every person brought a unique gift of friendship and care, but one gift in particular touched me deeply.

When the Oak Park congregation celebrated Stewardship Sunday in the spring, one of the adults in our congregation had offered a $1 bill to each of the young children, suggesting they spend the money for something they could later share with someone else. With his $1, Jesse bought flower seeds to be planted in the family's backyard. A colorful bouquet from Jesse graced the chancel for the memorial service. Ray would have been so pleased and I was too.

The children at church had discovered that if they stood close to Ray on Sunday mornings, he would gently massage their shoulders. He also enjoyed carving fanciful jack-o'-lanterns for the children at Halloween.

Pastor Ardean led in a meditation and a chaplain friend read Scripture; another played her guitar and sang. The words of condolence and encouragement were important, but most important to me was simply the presence of our friends. A warm handshake or a touch on the shoulder, a smile, a hug all communicated friendship, empathy, and love.

18

Heart-Wrenching Grief

The last memorial service was over. Tom and Carmen, Krista and Karen had returned to their homes. The defenses that had held me steady at first suddenly caved in, and I was filled with heart-wrenching grief. It affected every aspect of my life: physical, emotional, social, psychological, financial, and spiritual. The raw grief was a heavy weight on my chest. My voice was flat, lifeless. Often I awakened with a jerk in the middle of the night, only to realize that Ray was gone. Gone and never coming back. My psyche could not accept the finality of death in a single moment, day, month, or year. It was as if a new groove had to be worn into the brain and into consciousness before my psyche was able to adjust to the absence of the loved one.

Both my body and spirit were ready to collapse. However, there were too many details needing immediate attention to indulge the desire to collapse. New responsibilities rested on my shoulders: paying funeral expenses, ordering death certificates, changing the names on the bank accounts and the car title, paying the monthly bills, and filing the life insurance policies. Ray had always taken care of the finances, so reconciling the bank statement was a most intimidating task.

Each new chore reminded me that my life had changed radically—I was a widow. That was not an easy word to apply to myself after having been married for so many years. Gone were the days when one of us would drive around the block while the other ran into the post office or picked up something at the dry cleaners. All the household chores we had shared were now mine.

Many days I was aware of Ray's absence almost continually. Anywhere I turned in the apartment I found reminders of him. His chair across the table from me was empty, his closet full of his clothes. He was so present yet so absent. I found it comforting and painful to be in the space we had shared. A journal entry reflects such a day one week after the final memorial service.

This has been the toughest day yet. Most of the time I'm so aware that Ray is gone, gone, gone! Crazy as it may sound, one of his socks lay on his side of the bed, a symbol that this had been Ray's home. I leave it there all night to be near something that has belonged to him. I search for his wedding band and wear it to bed.

Tears can be healing, but they can be embarrassing when the dam breaks without warning, anytime, anywhere. I walked into a friend's woodworking shop one day to see about having him make a shadow box to hold some mementos. I approached the counter when unexpectedly tears began to stream down my face. This was not the time to explain what I wanted. I turned and left the shop without a word. On other days the tears were internal, pent-up in the lower abdomen.

The ability to concentrate had left me. When I most needed to think clearly to make sound decisions, the ability to do so was unavailable. Anger, which for years had been hidden under layers and layers of prohibitions, surfaced in the blink of an eye. My emotional fuse was especially short at even the slightest hint that someone might take advantage of me. I misplaced or forgot more things in a week than I care to remember. Financial concerns were frightening because my income would be considerably less than half of what our combined income had been.

God, so present during Ray's illness, seemed far away, unreachable. Often when I wanted to pray, there were no words, only a wordless crying out to God not to leave me alone in darkness and fear. I went to church but the joy and luster were missing. My voice was not trustworthy for either singing or speaking; the emotions were too close to the surface. I was grateful for friends willing to listen when I needed to talk and grateful to be included in social activities, just as the two of us had been included when Ray was still alive. From its beginning our little church was home for many singles and we had learned to include everyone in church activities.

Keeping a journal had been a useful way to pray and sort out priorities, gain new perspective, and maintain balance in my life for years before Ray's illness and death. Now writing became my primary form of prayer as I mourned. I was unable to concentrate long enough to engage in verbal prayer. My journal provided a safe way to explore and express my contradictory feelings of grief: loneliness, abandonment, anger, regret, guilt, blame, sadness, hope, love, and occasionally a hint of joy. I grieved for all I had lost, and for the loss of what never had been and never would be.

In early September, a month after Ray's death, I made arrangements to go to the Cenacle, a Catholic retreat center in Chicago. I planned to spend concentrated time working through my grief. Usually when I went to the Cenacle, I did not ask for spiritual guidance from one of the sisters; however, for this occasion I was eager for someone to give direction to my time there. The sister assigned to me met me in the lobby and showed me to my room. She invited me to make myself comfortable and said she would be available later in the evening if I needed her. In the meantime, she left me to relax alone. She had no more than closed the door when my defenses crumbled. Being in a safe place apparently sent a signal to my spirit, giving permission for my deepest grief to surface. I wept and wept. I felt like the tears might never end, but eventually they subsided. After the dinner hour I tried to reach the sister but was unable to locate her.

With no one to guide me, a new method to work through grief occurred to me. I decided to focus on memories and feelings associated with each room of the houses where Ray and I had lived: bedroom, bathroom, living room, kitchen, and family room. I began with the bedroom and wrote:

> The bedroom represents a place of rest and sleep. Often too tired for anything but quick kiss. Times of intimacy and pleasure and times of great frustration and disappointment. Something is wrong with me! I must be uninteresting and unattractive. The bedroom is the place where new life begins. Wonderful! Lying close when it was cold, warming my feet on his. Unexpressed anger. The place where Ray spent the last days of his life: iced tea, aspirin, sweats, fever, cool wet towels, where Ray's "little boy" came out to play—so beautiful! Crawling into bed with him, singing to him, caressing his burning chest. Now Ray is gone, his pillow vacant!

Through my journal I reentered a variety of memories—the painful and heartwarming, the big events and the trivial moments—to gradually integrate and claim more fully the life we had shared.

My work for the evening was not yet complete. I followed the journal writing with a visualization exercise. In my imagination Jesus stood on one side of our bed and I stood across from him. He invited me to take his outstretched hands; I placed my hands in his and together we thanked God for all that had happened in our bedroom and all it represented for me. Jesus and I blessed everything—pain, pleasure, disappointments, anger, and isolation—*everything*—for the deepening of my life. The work of the evening refreshed me and left me with new memories that could nourish my heart and spirit.

The following morning the sister suggested we walk through the neighborhood and spend time in Lincoln Park, one of my favorite places in all of Chicago. But I was miffed that she did not help me with my grief work and criticized her in my thoughts. Later I realized she had given me a gift by providing a break from the intensity of my emotions. Thus, I learned during my retreat that it is unhealthy to remain lost in grief full time. Working on memories associated with the rest of the rooms of the houses had to wait to be completed later. The sister and I met once more in the afternoon to bring closure to my time at the Cenacle. She suggested that I was feeling Ray's presence even since his death. That idea was foreign to me. What I felt was his absence! I had not expected to finish my grief work when I went to the Cenacle but was ready to leave with gratefulness for the sister and the work we had accomplished.

A year before Ray's death, I had attended a seminar on grieving. The seminar leader suggested putting into a box the special mementos that symbolized the person and the lost relationship. The idea was to set the box aside, bring it out periodically, and go through the contents in an unhurried manner, allowing into my awareness all the memories and emotions that surfaced. A second step was to acknowledge the memories and express the emotions in a tangible way. I intended to try the idea.

All the cards and letters Ray received during his illness and the cards and letters I received after his death went into my box. His 1984 appointment calendar with the names and telephone numbers of his gay friends, men in major cities all across the country wherever he had traveled, went into the box too. Was I being masochistic to include that book? I think not. I chose not to hide from the truth about Ray and his gay relationships. I was determined to include anything that could help me understand Ray as a gay man so that eventually he would become a whole person inside me, instead of the divided Ray I had known for so many years. I was convinced that the only way to heal from my agonizing grief was to leave nothing unexamined.

I listened to the audiotapes of the memorial services in Hesston and Oak Park. After inserting a tape into the hi-fi, I lay on the floor, listened, and wept as much as I needed to weep. Initially it was horribly painful, but I repeated the process until I was able to listen calmly and with gratitude as Ray's colleagues expressed their appreciation for his contribution to the nursing profession. I received great comfort, strength, and hope from the Scriptures, meditations, prayers, and music, of the memorial services. Repeated listening eventually brought warm memories of our many colleagues and friends in the faith community in Hesston as well as our fellow worshipers in Oak Park. I knew of no shortcut through the intense pain of acute grief, but I could choose to express the painful feelings rather than fleeing from them.

The movement of my grief, especially during the first year, was like walking along the beach at the water's edge. A wave may roll in gently, washing lightly over my toes and feet. The next wave arrives not quite so gently with the water reaching mid-calf. Then when my back is turned, a powerful breaker hits my hips with full force and almost knocks me to the sand. That was how I experienced my grief.

Loss and grief were not strangers to me even before Ray's death. My earliest memory is of the last few days of my paternal grandfather's life, of his funeral and his burial. I can still see the open grave, as my father held me in his arms. The coffin was lowered into the hole and the men shoveled the dirt into the grave. I remember hearing the thud thud of the dirt clods as they fell onto the coffin.

The impact of the death of my oldest brother at age thirty-two surfaced again. Our whole family had been devastated, yet the reality and finality of Sam's death had not seemed real to me for many months. My father died in 1969. I shed few tears during his funeral, telling myself that Dad was ready to go; he had lived a full life, his suffering was finally over. However, six months later during the funeral of an older man in our congregation, I found myself weeping profusely. In that moment I knew I was weeping for my father, not the man whose funeral was in progress. That memory helped me in my latest grief.

A second brother died after a ten-day illness at the age of fifty-one. He left a wife and four children. Again the shock was beyond any rational understanding. A year later the husband of my oldest sister died without warning, apparently of a heart attack. Joe had prepared the family's usual Saturday-evening rice and curry dinner. My sister found his body on the kitchen floor the next morning. I understood that all my losses were connected, but I needed to name them and keep them from becoming fused.

From these experiences, I had learned that death in our family had always been more than a family event; it had been a shared community event. The presence of friends and neighbors had provided support, encouragement, and comfort. I also reflected on my tendency to delay grieving. I understood and accepted it. The pain and loss of death is often too deep to begin immediately the necessary work of mourning.

I remembered the elective course I had taken during my first semester in seminary, "The Constructive Management of Grief." When reading the title, the word *grief* had resonated instantly. At last there was a name for the feelings associated with the deaths in my family, and with the losses of many familiar places and leaving many friends because Ray and I had moved our family so frequently. I registered for the course and gained a textbook knowledge of the necessary work of mourning to heal well from profound losses. I was very grateful that the course helped me understand the process of grieving, yet it could not diminish my pain.

During my seminary field education, my supervising chaplain had suggested I offer a seminar on loss and grief for a class of new nursing assistants at the hospital, and he also invited me to colead a weekly bereavement support group with him for the following year. People came to the weekly meetings as they felt the need for support. Members in the group taught me that feelings of anger, fear, depression, and guilt are triggered again and again by memories, thoughts, and experiences of daily life.

Neither the many deaths in my family of origin, my textbook knowledge of grief, nor listening to the pain and grief of others had fully prepared me for my plunge into grieving the death of my spouse.

New Year's Day 1985 arrived hard on the heels of Ray's death. Time was moving me away from his life much too quickly. I wanted to cling to the new openness we had created in the seven weeks following his diagnosis. Inwardly I cried again and again, Please just give us another chance to see what we can make of our marriage. It felt as if I were on a raft being carried out to sea, far from the shore and from the life I had lived with Ray, carrying me unrelentingly toward a distant shore that lay beyond the horizon.

My life was filled with so many conflicting thoughts and feelings. I was riding the emotional roller coaster again as I had during Ray's illness. I resisted the responsibility of making a living even though I was professionally well prepared to do so. I did not want to take care of others; I wanted someone to take care of me. I wanted to love and be loved. I wanted to be accepted as a woman. My feelings of yearning alternated with days of depression and despair. There were days when I was filled with rage, wanting to curse and swear. I was often angry with God. Why does God permit the terrible suffering in the world? An age-old question, yet it found an echo in my heart. A deeper awareness of our finite human limitations emerged as frustration.

My days of emptiness and the aching void induced emotional weariness far more severe than physical fatigue.

I wrote in my journal:

I've hit rock bottom! I don't want to go on, let me lie in bed, forget everything, cease to exist. What difference does it make what I do? Maybe I should get rid of everything and fall apart. Why keep trying?

The lament psalms fit my mood. I wrote a lament of my own:

Where shall I go?
There is no respite from the pain,
No escape from weariness.
I care nothing for work or friends.
Be quick! God,
save me before I end up in the grave.

19

A Gracious Interlude

When I signed a one-year contract as assistant director of field education with our denominational seminary in Elkhart, Indiana, I had no idea I would be a widow by the time I was to attend faculty retreat in late August. It was to be a trial year to see if the position fit my interests and skills with the option to stay long-term if I chose to do so. Three weeks after the memorial service in Oak Park, I joined the faculty on retreat in preparation for the new academic year.

One young woman, the wife of a faculty member, reached out to me during the retreat. To walk slowly and talk with this one person or be silent together was comforting. My pain was still too raw to meet and mix easily with the larger group of strangers, even though that too was part of the weekend. I felt alone amid a crowd. Returning to my home in Oak Park for several additional weeks before classes began was a great relief.

By the time classes began, I felt ambivalent about the commitment I had made. While I considered it a great privilege to be working with colleagues committed to serving the church, the new setting was another major change, another adjustment claiming my limited energy. A cardinal rule for the bereaved is to avoid major decisions and changes within the first year following the death of a spouse. But my decision had been made earlier, and I wanted to follow through with my commitment. Marcus (the former pastor I introduced earlier) was to be my supervisor. He had been in charge of field education for several years. I was to work four days a week during the trial year and commute weekly from my home in Oak Park.

Marcus and Dottie also invited me to live with them during my time in Elkhart. It was a gracious gesture that touched the depth of my heart. They expressed concretely what it means to be the church, members of the body of Christ. Joining others around their family table for meals nourished not only my body but also my spirit. They gave me a place to belong in a new family. Eating alone, I soon discovered, was one of the most difficult adjustments for me as a widow. Dottie, a hospice nurse, was sensitive to my needs, offering to listen if I needed to talk or sitting with me and gently rubbing my back. Her touch made her care tangible as I made the transition to living alone.

I considered my most important work for the year to be attending to my grief even though I also wanted to be responsible in my work. A few weeks into the new position, Marcus and I met in the office one evening for further orientation and to consider what was most important. After identifying matters needing immediate attention, Marcus shifted the focus to long-range planning. Suddenly I burst into tears. The outburst was as much a surprise to me as to him. "What happened?" he asked.

"I can't possibly think about long-range plans. All the energy I can muster is needed to accomplish the day-to-day tasks, one week at a time," I answered. Marcus paused, then suggested I return to my home the following morning and stay there until I felt able to return to work. To be offered that kind of understanding and flexibility was healing and reassuring.

The seminary had planned a weekend conference on sexuality to be held on campus in October. The final session was scheduled for Sunday evening to listen to the stories of a lesbian and a gay man with time for questions and discussion after their presentation. When I returned to Elkhart on Sunday evening, Dottie told me about the meeting on campus, and I decided to go. The group was small. During the discussion I said, "I would like to be part of a church where everyone—gay, lesbian, or straight—is welcome to worship together, simply accepting one another for who we are."

The next day a student called to schedule an appointment to see me. When we met his question was direct: "How does it happen that a woman your age expresses a wish that gay, lesbian, and straight people could all worship together in the same church?"

I said candidly: "My husband was a gay man and died of AIDS several months ago." I can still see his reaction to those words. He closed his eyes and sat quietly for a few moments, then spoke softly: "I have a brother who is gay." It was a freeing, grace-filled moment for me.

I appreciated learning to know the faculty and staff and working with students. I learned a great deal about the position and enjoyed my work as much as I could have enjoyed any work at the time. Chapel services were inspiring and refreshed my spirit. Without a doubt the greatest gift the faculty and staff offered me was space. No one probed or hovered; instead they accepted me with a warmth I found supportive.

Despite all the positive features of the work and the people at the seminary, it became clear that I needed to return to Oak Park to grieve fully. The friends I had known during my residency in Clinical Pastoral Education as well as the people in our church had known Ray and me as a couple. Ray was serving as the church administrator at the time of his death. In that position he led all congregational business meetings and served as chairperson of the church council. Many of these friends had extended their support during Ray's illness. People in the congregation grieved his hidden sexual life and tragic death. They were also angry and disappointed along with me. I felt safe with them. We had shared a history that could not be duplicated in a new environment. My need to return to Chicago became more and more urgent.

I remained at the seminary for sixteen months. By that time the seminary was able to find a person to fill the position. I will always be grateful for those sixteen months in which I caught a glimpse of the commitment, hard work, and excitement that is part of educating men and women for leadership in the church. It had been a healing, clarifying interlude touched by grace. That I had the opportunity to work at the seminary at all still seems to me nothing short of a miracle.

20

Complicated Grieving

The circumstances surrounding Ray's death complicated my grieving. Learning that Ray was gay was not a surprise—but that he had been sexually active, and lived secretly as a gay man for some years before his illness, shocked me to the core. It's true that we found new freedom to speak heart to heart once he had told me the truth about his diagnosis. That was like opening a window and breathing fresh spring air after spending years enclosed in a tightly sealed, suffocating room. But we had only a few short weeks to share the way each of us had experienced our life as marriage partners and as I struggled to understand what his life as a gay man was like for him. He was far too ill to engage in long conversations. Short snippets and vignettes were all we had. The greater impact of his disclosure surfaced little by little as the months of acute grief led into years of trying to make sense of what had happened.

I can only imagine the emotional stress he experienced as he revealed parts of himself that had been hidden and forbidden for so long. How I ached for him, for both of us, when I heard him saying, "I knew before we were married I was gay, but in those days there was nothing for a gay man to do but to marry and have a family. So that is what I did. As far back as I can remember, I knew I was different from other little boys. It was as a teenager that I discovered a name for what made me different from other young men. The impulse to know and explore my attraction to men became stronger and stronger as I grew older."

I found it impossible to grasp that what he was telling me applied specifically to him, to his life, to *my husband*. His words were clear enough, but the reality he described remained inconceivable to me. The images his words created were only dim, shadowy sketches, like the barely visible outlines of a painting, without clear definition. Surely, I thought, he is talking about a stranger. To tell the truth, I had often felt during the many years of our marriage that Ray was a stranger because he shared so little of his thoughts and feelings. Slowly, painfully, I decided to trust the journey, to grow in my readiness to claim our past and to embrace my future. God's transforming grace was always touching my life and at work within me.

As I considered what life might have been like for Ray knowing he was a gay man even before we were married, I realized he probably lived in torment. He must have been afraid his secret would be discovered, afraid of the shame, disgust, scorn, and rejection that would be directed at him by society, by the church, and perhaps even by members of his family. Several of his gay friends told me after his death that Ray was afraid he would lose me and our children if we were ever to discover his secret life. Ray knew the faith he had embraced as a young man considered homosexuality to be sinful above almost anything else.

More than a year after Ray's death I was grappling with issues I had not anticipated. A journal entry illuminates my quandary.

> Where is the thin line between accepting our pain as redemptive and dramatizing it? Sensationalism, exposure, high drama is not my style. Public property is not what I want to become. Being with people one-to-one or with a

few at a time is one thing; but I'm not sure how my ministry would be enhanced by greater publicity.

Ray, I don't know if you are aware of what I'm going
through. The betrayal, disbelief, the tortured grieving
and incongruity of my situation seems like a bad, bad
dream. It is no dream! Living through the two months of
your illness and the sixteen months since your death has
been the most intensely painful and concentrated struggle of my life. How so much change could be packed
into one year and four months is staggering.

Ray, do you understand that somehow I need you to
be the one out front? I need you to be saying, "Yes, I
want to stand in for Ann. I am the one who was gay. I
was afraid and I hid from myself, from her and, as much
as I could, from God. I was afraid to let them know who
I was. The cost seemed too great. I could not face the
possibility of losing Ann, my position, my reputation,
or my family. I was afraid and I hid.

"Today I stand beside her as she faces you and I say,
Let me speak. Let me speak for myself. Let me speak for
my brothers who are afraid and hide, those who hide
their fear in a way of living that becomes destructive. I
also speak for those who want desperately to be recognized as loving, lovable men. Men who want companionship, respect, acceptance and assurance that we are
like every other human with one exception—we love
men rather than women. Can't you hear our cry without
judging us?

"Ann, I love you even though our lives can never
again come together. I can't actually stand beside you.
You are the one whom I both loved and feared, feared
because every time I saw you, I was reminded I was hiding. I could not let you in close because you are strong
and made me feel inadequate. I want to stand beside you
as you walk Halsted Street and talk with gay men about
life and death."

Ray how do you feel about my being on TV? What will this do to the memories others have of you? If you were here would you sit beside me and say, "Yes, I have AIDS and I will die. I will leave a widow and four adult children. I will leave them trying to put together the pieces of their lives"? No, Ray I don't think you would do that. I don't have to do it either. I don't have to flaunt my strength, or my pain and weakness.

I am overwhelmingly sad, filled with loss and grief. I am sad that a life with so many gifts and talents was torn with so much love, alienation, desire, guilt, fear and, finally, the compulsion to risk everything for the sake of sexual pleasure, exploration, excitement, and adventure.

God, there is so much about life's ambiguity and complexity that I do not understand. I dare to offer my complaint before you because I have known you as a faithful God. Once more I bow before you in love, devotion, and surrender. Whatever the future holds, let your Spirit set me free to recognize the power of your love to discipline and to bring wholeness and redemption.

That Ray had lived a hidden life was such a blow because it was incongruent with the way he conducted the rest of his life, the life visible to others. He was upright and good. He was honest in his business practices, never cheating anyone out of a dime. He was conscientious in his work to a fault, generous in charitable giving, maintaining a discipline he had practiced before we were married. Ray was generous toward me in material things. Most of the beautiful things in our home were either gifts he had given me or things he had collected for beauty's sake. It was rare for him to be critical of the way I spent money. I had never known him to lie, yet after opening his secrets it was evident he deceived me many times during the latter years of his life.

I was outraged by his double life, and for him it was a great tragedy. His rejection and betrayal cut to the heart. I felt used and discarded as secondhand material, not valued as a woman. Anger became my familiar companion during my protracted grieving. There were times I wanted to hurt him as severely as he had hurt me. There were moments when I wanted revenge. Words that came flying out of my mouth describing my desire for revenge were a horror to me. I could hardly believe they had crossed my lips. I did not always protect Ray from my feelings of anger and betrayal although I did monitor my words carefully lest they should become destructive instead of facilitating healing.

Usually the vicious outbursts came when I was alone, in which case I found a close friend in whose presence I could safely express my venom. Often I turned the rage into words I committed to my journal, that dear and trusted soul friend. It was not only rage and rejection I wrestled with; I resented being thrust without choice onto a path that has tested me to the core and that shattered my basic notions about life. Again my journal reflects my disorientation.

> The framework of my life has been shattered, blown apart. I feel like I am in a foreign country whose terrain I never dreamed of traveling. It has been so easy in the past to say, "I couldn't make it without Christ," yet many people do. Or else Christ is present, holding all things together in a deeper way than is visible to the human eye.

I assumed that since God created us male and female, male-female marriage was God-ordained. Yet I had entered a male-female marriage that lasted more than thirty-one years, only to discover that my husband had been attracted to other men during all of those years. How was I to make sense of such a contradiction?

I had also assumed and expected that our common commitment to Christ—the foundation of our Christian marriage—and our vows of fidelity would create a bond that would lead us to know and trust each other completely. I had hoped our lives would be open to each other, creating both a spiritual and physical bond. Alas, I had not reckoned adequately with the wounds each of us brought into our marriage. My heart was broken as I realized both of us had fallen far short of our expectations and assumptions, short of our best intentions.

At the same time I felt convinced that God had not abandoned us in our failures, leaving us with nothing but pain and struggle. Instead God had remained faithful as we searched and stumbled around trying to find fulfillment in life. It was through the loving support of many friends and through personal spiritual disciplines that I gradually learned to rest in the gracious love that God extends to all of us in every circumstance and for all time.

How could it be that our marriage had been reduced to such chaos? I had spent inordinate amounts of time and energy trying desperately to create something of our relationship that proved impossible. Ray had fought for years to remain faithful to his marriage commitment, ultimately finding himself unable to sustain the battle to the end. I had been aware that homosexuality existed, and I had heard and read about infidelity in marriage but had no knowledge, no understanding, or inkling of the havoc that can invade and wreck a family when homosexuality and infidelity come together in a marriage. All these matters surfaced amid my grief. They intensified and confused the grieving process. But even more was at stake than complicated grieving. The confusion and conflicts raised serious theological questions for me. My inner urgency to explore these matters can hardly be overstated.

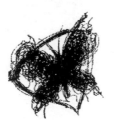

Part Four

Love is patient; love is kind; love is not envious or boastful or arrogant or rude. It does not insist on its own way; it is not irritable or resentful; it does not rejoice in wrongdoing, but rejoices in the truth. It bears all things, believes all things, hopes all things, endures all things.

—1 Corinthians 13:4-7

Love is what we do.

—Ann Showalter

21

A Search to Understand

Before Ray died I asked, "Are there gay friends who should be invited to your memorial service?"

"No, there is no one that close," he responded.

My heart caught in my throat as I thought, You are dying of an illness contracted through intimate contact, yet there is no one close enough to be invited to your memorial service. How tragic! I was not convinced it was true. Surely he was trying to protect me from further pain. I wanted to invite his friend Bill. I did not ask Ray's permission, but after his death I called Bill to notify him of the date and time of the memorial service in Oak Park. He was not at home when I called, so I left the message on his answering machine.

When I returned from the memorial service in Kansas, a letter from Bill was waiting for me. He said he would be out of town on business at the time of Ray's service and promised to remember him by attending church where he was going. He invited me to call him to go to lunch or dinner when I felt up to going out. I appreciated his proffered kindness.

The compelling urge to know Ray's gay friends emerged soon after his death. I wanted to be with people who had known him as a gay man. The compulsion was so clear and powerful that ordinarily I would have attributed it to God's

Spirit speaking to me. However, since it had to do with exploring something as new and foreign as learning to know my husband's gay friends, I wasn't sure it was safe to trust this particular urge. What if it was only curiosity? Or what if I was being tempted to go in a wrong direction? What if my exploration would lead me away from God? Despite the conflict, I pressed on. I could imagine no other way to understand and come to terms with the direction Ray had chosen in what turned out to be the last years of his life. I felt certain he had struggled with something very powerful, far more than a mere whim, for him to choose to live a hidden life. I hoped that in learning to know a few of his gay friends I would also learn to know him more fully.

I decided the least threatening place to begin was to get in touch with his physicians, who knew him in a professional capacity. The compassionate care Dr. David Blatt and Dr. David Moore extended to both of us was a significant factor in my decision to contact them. They were committed to providing the best medical treatments available at the time and to making their care as humane as possible.

I went to their office one afternoon, unannounced, to deliver a box of chocolates as a thank-you gift. The waiting room was full. I introduced myself to the receptionist, who told me Dr. Moore was out for the afternoon but let Dr. Blatt know I was waiting. Within minutes he invited me into his office, expressed his condolences, and said how sorry he and Dr. Moore were to have missed the memorial service. I was surprised and regretted I had failed to notify them. In my experience it was not customary for physicians to attend the memorial services of their patients. Later I learned these doctors did attend the memorial services of their patients. They wanted and needed a time and place to honor the memory of their friends and to grieve with their community. They considered the patients their brothers, and in the mid-1980s, patients with AIDS usually died within eighteen months to two years, often more quickly. Doctors become doctors because they want to save lives, but AIDS initially changed that possibility. It was exceedingly difficult to walk the path they were walking. I was in awe of their commitment.

I told Dr. Blatt my purpose in coming, thanked him for all they had done for Ray and me, and gave him the candy. He suggested I stop in again when Dr. Moore was in. I kept the visit short so he could get back with his patients.

Several weeks later I scheduled an appointment with Dr. Moore. We talked about Ray's illness and the support I had offered him. He said he had seen families who could not accept a son's sexual orientation or his illness and did not show compassion.

He asked if I would talk with other families trying to cope with the discovery that a son was gay and had contracted AIDS. It was not a difficult decision. I remembered the crucial role our friends filled as we lived through the wild fluctuations between Ray being close to death one day and seeing surprising improvements the next, even though these positive changes were usually of short duration.

"Take time to work through your grief until you are ready to relate to others, then call me and I will put you in touch with the person who brings family members and volunteers together," Dr. Moore said.

My fantasies told me Ray was probably a different person with his gay friends than with me. I imagined him to be uninhibited, sharing freely his interests, feelings, hopes, and fears. In mid-September, about six weeks after Ray's death, I called his friend Bill and let him know I was ready to go to dinner. He came to the apartment to pick me up at the appointed time, looked admiringly at the antique furnishings and said, "I didn't know Ray was into antiques." Bill had no idea how his comment affected me. He and Ray had dinner once a week, yet he knew nothing of Ray's interest in antiques. That certainly was not a threatening topic of conversation. Perhaps if Ray did not talk with his friends about a simple interest, they did not find him to be more free and open than I did.

My urge to know more about gay life extended far beyond Ray himself although it included him. I wanted to know and understand what it means to grow up gay or lesbian in the church and this culture. Young children and adolescents often become the targets of derogatory terms such as sissy, homo, half-and-half, fairy, faggot, queen, lesbo, and dyke. Beyond such negative name-calling are countless jokes with homosexual innuendoes, exaggerated mannerisms, and harsh condemnation from many pulpits. How do these messages affect gay and lesbian folk? Such comments do not create same-sex identity, but they isolate, alienate, and wound, often leaving them with a harsh inner critic, with self-denigration and self-hatred.

I scoured the library and bookstores for books about homosexuality. I read books on the causes of same-sex orientation, generally written by heterosexuals. It soon became apparent there is no consensus among scholars or theologians as to the roots of homosexuality. I read books on the effectiveness of psychotherapy and books on spiritual healing. I discovered it is not unusual for Christian heterosexual counselors to suggest exorcism for the gay or lesbian who is coming to the realization of his or her sexual orientation. I read books about gay life and relationships by gay authors.

One book, focusing on problems common to gay couple relationships, sounded as if it had been written for straight couples. The problems the author described were similar. They dealt with differences in personality and in ordinary likes and dislikes. Who was responsible for household chores, doing the laundry, cooking, cleaning? Who was to take care of the finances? Who decided how income was to be shared? What problems occurred when one person earned a larger salary than the other? How did the partner respond if one or the other suffers from severe depression or other illness? How did they negotiate when one person wanted more affection or desired more intimate contact than the other? All these problems are common to heterosexual marriages as well as to gay and lesbian couples. These are human problems rather than sexual-orientation issues.

I also discovered there are many problems unique to gay relationships, problems having more to do with public attitudes than with the relationships themselves. There is little public affirmation or sanction for gay and lesbian couple relationships. Public ceremonies to validate their commitments to each other are seen as inappropriate, undermining marriage. Everything from holding hands in public to looking for apartments, buying furniture, looking for employment, or shopping for groceries together makes couples easy targets for derogatory comments and being denied housing or employment. My primary question at the time was not whether gay relationships are right or wrong. Rather, I was looking for information and understanding.

Ray's friend Bill offered to help me in my search. He was a member of the Windy City Gay Men's Chorus. He invited me to one of their rehearsals and later to their Christmas concert at the People's Church in Chicago. The music was excellent but it was not the music alone that captured my attention. About 1,400 people were in attendance, fewer than fifty of them women. The numbers made a huge impact. I realized that homosexuality is not something found only in dark, hidden corners of big cities but in every community across the country. It had to be more prevalent than I thought possible.

Bill and I talked and talked, sometimes by telephone, at other times face to face. From our conversations and the reading I was doing, I soon realized that Ray's hidden life had no resemblance at all to the way either of us had been raised. It was clear that he had felt compelled to explore a part of himself he could not discover with me. Anger, compassion, empathy, and sadness were vying for places in my heart. A widening chasm separated what I believed with my intellect, including ideas I had internalized in my family and church, and what I was learning through my interaction with folk in the gay community.

My desire to understand the experience of gay men and women in our culture and in the church was not satisfied by learning about them from an objective distance or from a book. I wanted to learn what life is like for individual people, up close.

I reflected on the meaning incarnation has for me—God entering our world in the flesh-and-blood person of Jesus. As a human being Jesus knew human experience firsthand. He worked with his hands, did the hard physical labor of a carpenter. He knew hunger and thirst, fatigue and loneliness. He chose his closest friends from among those of little account by human standards. He was familiar with criticism and rejection and gladly received those whom the religious authorities considered unacceptable. In short, Jesus came in close. Are we who claim to be his followers not called to embody his Spirit in the world today? Did I have the strength and courage to begin a journey without knowing the outcome? By God's grace, yes. I wanted to come in close, I wanted to listen and learn directly from those consigned to the margins by mainstream society and the church.

I was convinced I had to listen without immediately quoting the Scriptures used to condemn homosexuality if I wanted to understand the experience of gay and lesbian folk. Therefore I decided to put those Scriptures on a shelf, so to speak, and simply listen and learn. My role was not to bring dos and don'ts or shoulds and should nots but to be present to each person whose life touched mine.

The decision to put Scriptures on a shelf did not mean I no longer had access to them; it meant I would not use them to defend a personal stance. I soon discovered it was more painful to listen without defense than to quote Scripture. I saw how easy it is to employ Scripture as armor to protect oneself from the raw pain and inner struggles of a fellow human being. Using Scripture to defend myself would have put distance between us. It would have created a space in which I could have felt safe while leaving the other person isolated. There are times when offering Scripture is appropriate, but my first purpose was to listen and learn. Without the armor, trust developed quickly, and I soon heard the real stories of gay men I met.

I was often scared of the journey because I did not know where it would lead. I worried about compromising my faith because of messages I had internalized in the past. My questions sent me again and again to look carefully at the life of Jesus. For me, his relationships are the consummate pattern, and I see Jesus' life as the ultimate interpretation of Scripture. I found that Jesus reached out freely to people whom the religious authorities, for a variety of reasons, rejected as unworthy. The Jesus of the Bible was open to anyone open to receiving him. I also rediscovered that the religious leaders became the targets of Jesus' harshest criticism, not because he did not love them but because of their lack of compassion.

To complicate matters even more, I remembered vividly that it was the ministry of a gay priest that had touched me with grace, hope, and a measure of healing before Ray's illness. I felt compelled to ask, Does God, then, work in and through people whom the church, for the most part, rejects? I examined the lives of the patriarchs and matriarchs of the Old Testament. All of them had major human flaws, yet God chose them to accomplish God's purposes.

What about the doctors who had provided such compassionate care for Ray and me? What is the origin, the source of such compassion? Who was Jesus talking about in Matthew 25 when he invited into the Father's presence those who had ministered to the "least of these" without recognizing they were offering service to God? I was not sure what to make of my search. These were serious, troubling questions with which I wrestled without finding quick resolution for them. They circulated through my mind and heart over and over, demanding recognition, demanding my answer. The depth of my frustration with the troubling questions is reflected in another journal entry.

> Lord, I did not ask to be thrust into this turmoil! Now I am overwhelmed, battered on every side. The outward circumstances cry for compassion, yet my heart is torn by fear. I fear aligning myself with people who do not call for repentance to follow Christ; they speak and live with compassion instead of obeying rules and commandments.

Many Christians insist they love and are open to persons of same-sex orientation; but to be received into the church, gays and lesbians must first repent of their "sin" and forgo their needs for intimacy. I understood that kind of thinking well, for it had been mine until I began my impassioned exploration. I remember the day a gay minister explained that often the gay or lesbian person must first of all repent of instilled self-hatred and self-denigration to discover that God loves and receives him or her into a loving relationship. His comments were penetrating, worthy of further reflection.

22

The Imperative
to Embrace

Eight months after Ray's death, I felt ready to reach out to others who knew firsthand the shattering effects of losing a loved one to AIDS. I remembered Dr. Moore's invitation to let him know when I was ready. I called him. He suggested I call Tim, the director of volunteers, at Howard Brown Memorial Clinic on North Halsted Street, a health-care clinic with gay men as the primary clientele. I contacted Tim, and he sent me an application that was extensive and thorough. I completed the application and returned it. After evaluating the information, Tim called me to schedule a personal interview. The men who came and went as I sat in the waiting area to be called for my appointment glanced at me from the corner of their eyes. It was obvious that few women with gray hair frequented the clinic.

Tim was amiable as we discussed my resume and the skills I could bring. He was especially interested to note that I had previous experience in working with grief support groups. He asked if I would be willing to lead such a support group for gay men. I was interested and said so without hesitation. Tim asked a few questions related to the culture and lingo of the gay community. Because of my reading I was familiar with the matters he raised and able to respond satisfactorily.

We set a time and place for me to meet with the first group. We gathered in a room at the clinic on Easter Sunday afternoon. Ten men showed. It was no surprise that the conversation was guarded initially. To speak candidly with a complete stranger about personal loss and grief requires a great deal of vulnerability.

At one point I said, "You must be thinking, 'Who will be next?' "

"No," someone responded, "not *who* will be next, but will *I* be next?"

What a difference in perspective! Change one word and the possibility of who may be next becomes personal.

Before our meeting was over, I said, "Now I am going to take off my facilitator's hat and become part of the group. I know something about the loss and grief AIDS leaves in its wake. My husband died of AIDS about eight months ago." Instantly we were no longer strangers but members of a family of grieving people largely hidden from the general public and the religious community. At once I realized how privileged I was to be part of a church community that was supportive of my journey, while the church is the last place the men in this circle could go to for support. Even now I want to weep because it is still so for most people in the gay community.

One man in the group—once married to a woman—asked about my experience of being married to a gay man. As I described what life had been like for me, several times he said, "That's just what my wife said." I fail to find words that adequately describe my feelings as I heard for the first time of another woman who had shared my feelings, even though we had never met. My experience had been validated.

Soon it became apparent these men knew the pain of living with a secret, even as Ray and I had known. Through my bereavement work, I became convinced that the need for secrecy makes gay men more vulnerable to acting out their sexual desires in harmful ways. The need for secrecy intensifies the feelings, which leads to greater urgency to act upon the feelings. They look for moments of comfort to relieve their fear and the resulting tension.

Where were people of same-sex orientation to go for support and understanding? One young man told me how tired he was of the whole bar scene, yet there were few places he could safely go to find support, care, and companionship.

Protecting his secret ultimately led Ray to living a secret life, but I too had been affected by the secret because it *remained* a secret. There had been few people with whom I felt safe enough to even think of sharing my growing suspicion that Ray might be a gay. Maybe I was reluctant to speak with others about my suspicion because I was not ready to examine what it might mean for our marriage if I knew that Ray was gay.

A second reason to keep my hunches to myself was that no one in the straight community, with the exception of professional counselors, talked about same-sex relationships in the 1960s and 1970s. The "coming out" of the gay community, in the sense that it became politically active and thus initiated its own civil rights movement, did not occur until 1969. The men in the bereavement group understood my sense of isolation like few people in the straight community could have understood. Their responses after I revealed my husband's death from AIDS were a gift of grace.

The group that had gathered on Easter Sunday afternoon soon thinned out. Grief work is difficult and painful, especially when the participants are asking, "Will I be next?" During that summer we changed the meeting time to a weekday evening. Often only a few men showed and occasionally only one.

I remember the evening one man came alone. His facial expression, the pain in his eyes, and the slump of his shoulders as he sat facing me all spoke of sadness. He wept and said, "It feels like the gay community is being singled out for a terrible plague. Are we guilty? Are we being punished? Do we deserve this plague of AIDS?" He was his own harsh judge, reflecting

the self-hatred many gay people internalize, at least in part, because of the derogatory messages they hear from society and especially from the church. It was common for pastors and radio
or TV evangelists to make pronouncements that AIDS was
God's punishment on the gay community for a sinful lifestyle.
I suggested to this young man that God suffers with us when we
suffer, that if Jesus were alive, he would be walking Halsted
Street (an area with a large gay population) with a message of
compassion. Continuing to weep, he said, "If only I could believe that, I could make it."

Often such a conversation generated in me enormous internal conflict. Two inner voices, each reflecting sincerely held
convictions, carried on intense conversations. I knew that anyone suffering the devastating effects of AIDS deserved compassionate care. Furthermore, compassion came spontaneously
when I was face-to-face with these who were suffering. It was
later, when I was alone, that a second voice clamored to be
heard. The internal argument went something like this:

> *You know that you have a great responsibility to give witness*
> *that Jesus died for our sin. You are not speaking clearly*
> *about repentance and Jesus' love so that someone can know*
> *how to receive Jesus into his life if he wants to.*

But actions speak louder than words.

> *How can you be sure your desire to show the kind of com-*
> *passion Jesus showed is adequate? Who do you think you*
> *are? What about your decision not to quote Scriptures used*
> *to condemn homosexuality? How can that be right?*

When I refuse to use Scripture to defend myself, trust is
established. The questions and conversations sometimes
feel relentless.

The fact that I was a clergyperson willing to listen, learn,
and try to understand was not lost on people. The depth of

warmth and acceptance accorded me by people affected by AIDS spoke to me of the alienation they experienced from many in the institutional church.

One evening in 2002, I went upstairs for bed after spending hours writing. It was late, and I knew I had to unwind before I could sleep. As I passed my bookcase in my bedroom, I pulled from the shelf *Bread for the Journey*, a book of daily meditations by Henri J. M. Nouwen. I turned to the reading for the day but saw it was related to that of the previous day. I turned back one page, and this is what I read: "To be a witness for God is to be a living sign of God's presence in the world. What we live is more important than what we say, because the right way of living always leads to the right way of speaking."[2] I was amazed. It was a resounding confirmation of the lonely path I had chosen to follow in my ministry. What could I do but give thanks in worship and prayer?

My journal became a safe avenue to organize my thoughts, to wrestle into clarity what was confusing and regain perspective. Our congregation in Oak Park was a source of nurture, inspiration, and affirmation. My monthly visit with my spiritual guide was another resource that refreshed and strengthened me. Paradoxically, there was mutuality in my ministry to those affected by AIDS, including the bereaved, since many of them ministered to my spirit as I ministered to theirs. My work with the bereaved especially helped my healing. People in the bereavement groups usually were healthy or HIV positive. As I listened to the anguish of person after person, it became clear that gay men are as familiar with the complex emotions associated with grief—sadness, disappointment, fear, guilt, and anger—as any of us in the straight community. We all share a common humanity. Later I will address factors that made grieving AIDS-related deaths especially difficult.

23

Going Outside the Gate

In the twenty months after Ray's death, I had read numerous books, helped bereavement groups, connected with some of Ray's friends, and listened to many personal stories. The time had come to look for someone to guide me through the chaos and confusion, the turmoil and torment of my heart. Over the years I had spent a great deal of time in therapy, which had been beneficial, but I was through with that for the time being. I was ready for someone to help me delve into theology, the meaning of suffering, and what it means to follow Jesus in daily life. I contacted a seminary professor I had met through a friend and asked if he would become my spiritual director. He agreed to talk with me after the spring term ended.

In our first meeting I told him about Ray's illness and death and what I wanted. By the end of the conversation we both decided we could work together. Over the next four and a half years he spent many hours listening patiently to my questions, making observations and occasional suggestions that opened new vistas of faith for me.

One of the great gifts he offered was a suggestion to explore the journey of Abraham as a paradigm for my work with AIDS. I read and reread all of the Abraham stories looking for analogies. I found much that correlated with my work. The invitation to leave a safe, familiar "homeland" to follow a "calling" into AIDS ministry was like setting out on a journey into a new country. The landscape was rough and fearful, largely unexplored except by medical experts, and even the experts were in new territory. AIDS ministry called for willingness to explore a different culture and a new language as I prepared to offer AIDS education. Knowing and talking comfortably about blood platelet counts, immune deficiency, and T-cells and describing how HIV is transmitted in terms that even a high school student could understand had not been part of my experience. Becoming familiar with the host of infections common to AIDS was another kind of strange territory. Like Abraham, I discovered that God was present in places I would not have expected (see Gen. 20:1-11).

My friend and guide also suggested a brief passage from the book of Hebrews that I found fit my work. Most often we in the church remain safely within boundaries we have established between those who are "inside" and those who are "outside." The author of Hebrews writes: "For the bodies of those animals whose blood is brought into the sanctuary by the high priest as a sacrifice for sin are burned *outside the camp*. Therefore Jesus also *suffered outside the city gate* to sanctify the people by his own blood. *Let us then go to him outside the camp and bear the abuse he endured*" (Heb. 13:11-13, emphasis added). In the eyes of many people in the church, ministry to people with HIV/AIDS was neither a safe nor a desirable place to be. Working with men and women affected by AIDS meant going "outside the gate" because the church for the most part had been content to remain safely within the sanctuary.

A series of stories from my files provides a glimpse of what it meant for me to go outside the gate. These accounts highlight a number of particularly painful issues common to people with AIDS and those who loved them.

Kevin Is Not Ray

The door to the hospital room was open. I entered the room quietly and approached the bedside. A man I will call Kevin lay in bed with eyes closed. Perhaps he was asleep? Or was he comatose? His face, arms, and hands were covered with Kaposi's sarcoma, a cancer of the tiny blood capillaries, except for the back of his left hand. I reached across the bed railing, took his left hand into my mine.

"Kevin, my name is Ann. I'm a chaplain and came by to be with you for a little while."

There was no response, not a flicker of an eyelid or the raising of an eyebrow to indicate awareness. I sensed that it was no time for words, presence was enough. I held his hand for a half hour, not knowing whether he was aware of anything. Then out of the silence came his quiet words, "Your hand feels so good." Five simple words that touched my heart, for they conveyed so much about aloneness and presence and communion.

AIDS was a new and terrifying disease. People were afraid: afraid of the disease, afraid to come close to the person, and afraid to touch. This vignette became a metaphor for all the people I met during more than six years of working with those directly affected by HIV/AIDS, whether they were the ill or lovers, partners, friends, or family members. My desire was to be present, accept, and touch—whether physically, emotionally, or spiritually. I wanted to come close.

I left Kevin's room to go about my work for the rest of the day with no awareness of being depressed even though he was in the same room my husband had occupied just before being discharged to go home for the last days of his life.

The following morning I awoke to feeling something heavy on my chest. I knew instantly I had taken Kevin's pain into myself during my visit the previous day. What was I to do? As pastoral care coordinator for a hospice team, I knew I would meet other patients with AIDS. I was afraid of becoming immobilized if I carried their pain within me.

A day or two later I was thinking about Kevin as I drove to-ward my work in Elkhart, Indiana. I talked audibly to myself. "Ann, Kevin is not Ray. It is sad he is dying of AIDS, but his death will not affect your life as Ray's did. You will not be re-sponsible for the tasks you were responsible for when Ray died. You will not be ordering death certificates or filing insurance claims." On and on I talked to myself until I became clear who was suffering. Kevin was not Ray.

As long as I remained clear that the person suffering was not Ray and therefore would not affect my life as Ray's death had, I was free to be present to people with AIDS, without tak-ing their pain into myself. It proved to be a crucial discovery.

One Woman's Lament

Mary lived some distance from Chicago but came to visit her son. She was the mother of four sons. One had died young because of a congenital heart condition. A second son had been sent to Vietnam and did not return alive. All she had left of him were her memories, perhaps some medals, a grave, and an American flag.

"My coworkers, my neighbors, and friends at church were all supportive during those two losses," she said. "So when my third son was stricken with AIDS, I told my colleagues, neigh-bors, and friends at church what was happening. Now, *nobody* asks, 'How is your son?' or, 'How are you?'"

Isolation was like a cruel curse inflicted on a family when a son or daughter contracted AIDS. The isolation reached into all the tender places of the heart and seared its imprint into the spirit. I wonder if the pain of Mary's isolation still infects and sullies the precious memories of her son.

A Mother's Fear

My office telephone rang. It was a request to visit a young woman in a suburban hospital. She sat up in bed to tell me the following story:

After being tired and weak for many months, she visited her doctor in a rural area of the state. He was unable to discover the source of her problems, even though she saw him repeatedly. Eventually he referred her to a physician in suburban Chicago, where she was admitted to the hospital. She had undergone a whole battery of tests, and still the source of her problem eluded the doctor. Finally, the patient herself asked if it was possible that her fatigue could be related to HIV infection, whereupon the doctor ordered a screening test for HIV. The result was positive.

She was devastated, tormented, terrified. What was she to tell her husband, her children, her pastor, or the extended family? She had young school-age children. "Who will care for them when I am no longer able to care for myself or them? How will they remember me when I'm gone? How can I ever tell anyone the truth?

"I feel like a hypocrite for lying to the pastor and the people at church. But I'm scared of what might happen to the children if anyone ever discovered the truth." She had been lonely and had a fling while her husband was away from home on government business for many months.

This mother did not fit the perceived profile of a person at risk for HIV, hence the long delay in the diagnosis. It happened over and over. The denial went like this: AIDS is a disease of white gay men or of drug addicts or of a particular ethnic group—the disease was always perceived as the curse that belonged to someone else. It would be years before people faced the truth that the virus that destroys the immune system is incapable of choosing whom to infect and whom to pass by. Anyone who engages in the behaviors that transmit the virus is at risk for developing the infection.

Alone and Afraid

Sam approached my office for the first time, shy and soft-spoken.

"I'll take your coat and hat," I offered.

"Thank you."

He waited to sit down until I invited him to do so. Sam's head was shaved as smooth as a baby's bottom, not even a hint of fuzz. His head was nicely shaped, no bony lines or knobs.

"I like your bare head, it is actually quite handsome."

"Thank you," he said. For a moment, I saw a spark of light in his eyes.

I had no illusions that Sam was modeling the latest hair(less) fashion in the gay community. Chemotherapy was the culprit. Sam was not particularly tall or strongly built, yet he had a nice body. His eyes were brown wells, filled with pain. They glistened with tears from time to time as he drew out his story, painful word by painful word, a tortured process.

"I am going to die and am so afraid of being left alone. Maybe if I go home my family will care for me. We will have to build a relationship that has never really existed. I have never felt like I fit in, alone even when I lived at home. My folks don't know I'm gay. I did tell my brother and his wife."

I saw Sam several more times. During one of those visits, he told me he was considering suicide. After further conversation he made the decision to go home to his family, hoping they would receive him and care for him.

Sam's struggle was a common one when a young person discovered she or he was infected with HIV. Often the person could not imagine telling the family he was gay or that she was a drug user or had been infected by a husband who used drugs. It was too much to reveal in one fell swoop, too much for a family to hear in one fell swoop.

I Want to Be Free

I never knew what to expect when I answered my telephone in the office. A nurse I knew called to ask if I would go to the bedside of a friend of his. The friend wanted to talk about end-of-life issues. The request was out of the ordinary, since I usually had the opportunity to meet the person before needing to address those issues. It was a signal that this man was probably very ill and nearing the end of his life.

I went to the hospital and found Charlie wearing an oxygen mask to ease his breathing. He was pale, his face gaunt and his eyes deep-set, signs of the late stages of AIDS.

"Good afternoon. I'm Ann Showalter, I understand you wanted me to make a visit."

"Yes, thank you for coming." His voice was weak and he spoke slowly.

"I read recently of a man in another state who requested that after his death his ashes be put into 350 helium balloons and be set free. That sounded so wonderful. I want to be set free like that. Would you put my ashes into helium balloons and set them free?"

His request took me off guard because it was so out of the ordinary. I maintained my composure and said, "Yes, I'll do that for you." I stayed at the bedside for a few minutes before asking, "Is there anything else I can do for you?" Honoring his initial request had opened the door to further conversation.

"I wonder if I'm being punished," he said sadly.

"If you mean is God punishing you with AIDS, the answer is no. However, we sometimes make choices that have consequences we did not expect and could not foresee. When that happens we can always come to God and ask forgiveness. Would you like me to pray with you?"

He nodded.

As I prayed, the tears streamed down his face. We said our good-byes, and I left.

A day or two later, the nurse friend called again: "Charlie has been discharged from the hospital and is going home to the apartment to die. His partner is there to care for him, and they want to know if you would stop by the apartment on your way home." He gave me the address.

I went to see them on my way home that afternoon. Charlie's partner invited me to their upstairs apartment.

"My mother and sister are coming from out of state to visit on Saturday morning," Charlie said. "Would you come meet with us? I would like you to tell them what I want done with my ashes. Would you do that?" (Sometimes family members who had been distant during the illness showed up after death with their plans for the funeral and burial. Charlie did not want that to happen.)

"I'll be glad to come and talk with them."

As I prepared to leave, Charlie asked, "Will you pray with us before you leave?" We held hands as I prayed.

Saturday morning came, and I went to the apartment once more. His mother and sister were not present in Charlie's room when I arrived. Charlie and his partner and I had the opportunity to visit for a few minutes before his mother and sister joined us. After introductions I told them what Charlie wanted done with his ashes after his death. "I have promised to see that his wishes are honored." They offered no resistance, nor did they make counter suggestions. We took time to get acquainted before I prepared to leave. Charlie's lover was sitting in bed with him.

"Will you pray with us again?" Charlie asked. We all joined hands, mother and sister included, and I prayed a farewell prayer with them.

When Charlie died, his nurse friend notified me. "Ann, several of his friends and I will see to putting his ashes into the balloons." It was their last gift to Charlie, and it seemed appropriate to me that they wanted to take responsibility for fulfilling Charlie's last wish. They stopped at 125 balloons because of how tedious it was to get just the right amount of ashes into each balloon. Too many ashes and the balloons would not fly.

I met with several of Charlie's friends to plan the memorial service and later led the service and gave the homily. We left the church a little after sunset, each person holding the strings to a cluster of balloons as we made our way to the nearby shore of

Lake Michigan. The colorful balloons were tugging at the strings as if eager to be on their way. We stood together on the beach, remembering Charlie, and set the balloons free. It was a beautiful sight, an awesome moment touched by grace.

Charlie's request symbolized the deep longings of many in the gay and lesbian community "to be free." To feel the need to guard secret lives for reasons of safety or to avoid the risk of rejection by family, the church, and society is the antithesis of freedom.

♣

Each person had a unique story, and the progression in which the illness unfolded was unique as well. During the early years of HIV/AIDS, many people died within a few months of a diagnosis of full-blown AIDS. When I was working with a hospice team, one of our nurses was on duty one week, caring for patients as usual, and the next week I conducted *his* memorial service.

The response of family members when they discovered a son or daughter had contracted AIDS was as unpredictable as the disease itself. Their shock, fear, anger, or acceptance of the person was expressed in a variety of ways. Some responses were beautifully tender and loving while others were heartrending beyond words.

"Let us then go to him outside the camp to bear the abuse he endured."

24

The Power of Fear and the Power of Compassion

The stigma and shame associated with AIDS have presented a challenge for communities of faith as few other crises in recent history have done. Two major taboos—sex and death—converge in AIDS to create serious barriers to a compassionate response. The intense suffering of people affected by HIV/AIDS cried out (although no voice was heard) for communities of faith to become places of compassion and healing. Too frequently the response was silence, fear, and hostility. Occasionally a few were moved to compassionate action.

Today, more than twenty years after AIDS first appeared on the scene in this country, it is almost impossible to recapture the pervasive fear that was present in every stratum of society. I will long remember the statement of a mother who traveled several hundred miles from another state to Chicago to visit her seriously ill son. "If my friends at home knew I had a son with AIDS, I would lose my job," she reported. Whether or not she actually would have lost her job, I cannot say. I do know people often reacted as if the virus could be transmitted casually through a handshake or washing hands at the same sink or from a hug. Being told that the virus was transmitted only in specific ways was not enough to allay the fear. The fear was insidious and decidedly more contagious and more readily transmitted than the virus that destroys the immune system.

I certainly did not make light of the seriousness of AIDS; it was and is a dreadful, destructive, and ugly disease, particularly frightening because there is no cure. But the shame and stigma carried a huge load of freight as well. Those of us living in the United States had lived in a society that tried to deny the reality of death. Usually the dying were consigned into the hands of professionals, either in hospitals or nursing homes, and after death they were buried by professionals. Seldom was death allowed in close. Our society had developed the illusion in the thirty or forty years before HIV infection that medical science was "god." People who were ill expected, even demanded, a cure for everything. Such denial of death is primarily a phenomenon of Western industrialized society. People in most countries of the world know death to be as much a part of everyday life as birth.

Into this denial of death and the illusion of human control came a microscopic invader that stripped away our illusions, displayed our vulnerability, and ruthlessly confronted us with our human limitations. People were terrified. Those of us who worked with the ill and dying were not immune to fear but had to confront it if we wanted to work effectively with people.

Fear was especially poignant for parents from small-town U.S.A., for whom a large city was itself a frightening place. Add to that receiving in a single phone call information that their son was gay and seriously ill with AIDS, and a family could easily feel overwhelmed. Parents sometimes came to the hospital too frightened to do more than step inside the room. Coming close enough to offer a touch or a hug was out of the question. Often they were haunted by what they had done "wrong" to have raised a gay son. A mother could imagine that it was "caused" because she had not breast-fed or perhaps she had allowed the toddler to play with a sister's dolls.

It seemed unfair to attribute such fear to a lack of feeling or concern or acceptance of the person. More likely the distance between the life experience of the parents and the life experience of the person with AIDS was simply too great. There was no safe bridge across the chasm that separated one from the other. The image for me was that of expecting someone to step from the bottom rung of a ladder all the way to the top rung in one giant step. It could not be done.

I also met parents whose love and internal strength was such that they embraced the son or daughter and shared in their terrible dilemma of suffering. They lived with the agony of knowing that the life of their beloved adult child would ebb away too early. Despite—or perhaps because of—that awareness, they chose to move into the city temporarily to care for their loved one.

Two stories illustrate opposite poles on a continuum of response.

We Cannot Come!

The young man in Chicago was dying of HIV-related illness. His condition was deteriorating rapidly. A hospice nurse called his family in another state to let them know their son was seriously ill. No one came to visit. The following week the nurse called again to say that, if the parents wanted to see their son alive, they needed to come immediately. "We are Christians," they said; "we do not approve of his lifestyle. We cannot come!" The young man died without receiving the love of his parents and without the opportunity to say good-bye. The faith of the parents did not allow them to reach out to their own flesh and blood in compassion. Even parental love could not move them beyond their controlling prohibitions.

Anger and compassion struggled for first place in my heart when I heard the story. My own internal conflicts, frequent as they were, did not prevent me from feeling judgmental toward those parents. (I mean that as confession.) Yet I cannot fathom turning away from my own dying child.

Compassion

Amilia, a young woman with AIDS, no longer required hospitalization although she was not able to completely care for herself. Her family, with younger children at home, was not willing for her to come home to live until her death. Other than hospitals, there were no care facilities available for women with AIDS at the time. A nurse who had cared for her in the hospital, after talking over the situation with her husband and daughter, invited Amilia to live with her family. Amilia's life expectancy was two to three months at the most.

Soon after moving in with her new family, Amilia prepared a Puerto Rican dinner for them one evening. That did it. The husband became an immediate fan of Puerto Rican food. Since her hostess continued her work in the hospital, Amilia often cooked for the family when she was physically able. There was love, acceptance, and work to do. Life had meaning and purpose once more. Amilia lived for ten months. The family had put their faith into action and shared their love and compassion. They found joy and satisfaction in their friendship with Amilia, and she found hope and meaning.

Weakness Surrounds Me[3]

Weakness surrounds me,
I fear my aloneness. When
will you come to me, Lord? Wipe
away my fears, comfort my longing,
nurture my broken heart and save me from myself. . . .
Guide me in your light, raise me
from my death—this living hell
in which I dwell.

Purge my soul that I may walk
in Thine eyes
and perceive the vision
of your glory.
Break the mask of falseness
we have forged from disgrace—
and with Thy holy love,
replace. Teach us the way
Lord Jesus Christ, heal
our disease and strip us
of our perversity.
Take me tonight, Lord,
recast me in Your Light.
Heal me and set me in Your path
for I have gone
astray and I have utterly
lost who I am. Cast me
from the darkness.
You created me to walk
in this form, please
do not abandon me in this God-forsaken land.
—*Edward Byrnes Riley*

25

A Vision Is Born

Father Jim Corrigan, a chaplain supervisor in the Clinical Pastoral Education department at Rush-Presbyterian—St. Luke's Medical Center, was sitting across the table from me over lunch. His tone of voice and the energy with which he spoke betrayed his excitement. Jim and a number of his clergy friends had been providing pastoral care for persons with AIDS (PWAs) they met in their ministries and volunteer work. However, the larger task of providing spiritual support to PWAs throughout the Chicago area was much too large for a few people to undertake. Many of their gay brothers were suffering and dying without the healing benefit of pastoral care. Jim and his colleagues were determined to do what they could to fill that gap. They also knew that if those affected by AIDS were to receive compassionate care, the care would have to be rooted in the gay community.

Those in the core group shared their vision with others, inviting them to meet monthly to brainstorm, educate themselves about AIDS, raise funds, and form a board of directors with people committed to the unfolding vision. A group of specially trained volunteers appeared to be the best way to enlarge the circle of pastoral support.

Suddenly Jim's eyes lit up. "It just occurred to me that you are the person to become the coordinator of pastoral care when we are ready to employ staff," he said. He made it clear that he had no authority to offer me a position since the organization was still in its early stages.

It was my turn to be excited. I was working two part-time jobs, one of which would end within six months. Nothing else was in sight; so even though Jim's word was not a promise the possibility gave me hope.

The possibility Jim suggested was especially welcome at the time of our conversation, since my work at the seminary in Elkhart would be ending within six months. My second part-time position was that of pastoral care coordinator with a hospice team through Illinois Masonic Hospital. I was also continuing my volunteer bereavement work with Howard Brown Clinic. At the time all the bereavement work was with individuals. The possibility of another paid position was truly a word of hope even though I did not know how long it would be until the new organization Jim spoke of would be ready to hire staff. From August 1984 when Ray died and I began my work at the seminary until October 1986 my professional life was like a mosaic—one small piece after another fitting together.

About a year after that first luncheon conversation, Jim invited me to submit my resume to the board of directors of the AIDS Pastoral Care Network (APCN). I did so, and by the time I met with the board for an interview, they had recruited Father Carl Melrose as executive director for the organization. I was offered and accepted a half-time position as director of pastoral services. With less than $20,000 in the treasury, this was a venture of faith for all of us.

Carl and I began our employment on October 1, 1986. My bedroom at home became my first office. I realized when I accepted the position that I was in new territory. Although my husband had died of AIDS and I had provided bereavement support for gay men, to be employed by an *interfaith* organization with its roots in the *gay community* was a stretch for my Amish and Mennonite soul. It meant my work would become public, and I was not entirely comfortable with that. My volunteer work had been much less visible, virtually unknown in religious communities in the Chicago area or within my own faith tradition, with the exception of my home congregation in Oak Park. Accepting the position with APCN changed all that. My ministry became a public ministry.

Jim's first suggestion that there might be a place for me in the new organization was good news, but my decision to accept the position came only after considerable thought and prayer. There were no role models except for the compassion, understanding, and acceptance of Father Corrigan and the compassionate care of Dr. Moore and Dr. Blatt.

Carl was taking a walk in his neighborhood one evening and noticed that several floors of a Lutheran hospital were dark, as though unoccupied. He promptly wrote a letter to the hospital administrator about our ministry and our need for office space. He followed the letter several days later with a phone call. In a matter of days the hospital had granted APCN adequate office space and basic office furniture, all of it rent-free. We were elated.

The board of directors met with Carl and me in mid-October to set the direction for our ministry. At the end of the day we had designated four areas of ministry to guide us: (1) education, (2) direct pastoral care, (3) spirituality, and (4) public relations and development. Since Carl was responsible for the fourth area, I am not in a position to write about that aspect of our ministry.

I cannot imagine anyone filling that position with more grace, greater expertise, or in a manner more pastoral than Carl. He was an effective liaison between APCN and other AIDS service providers. One of my great joys during my five years with the network was working closely with Carl.

There was considerable overlap within the four areas of APCN's ministry. Initially Carl and I worked together in our educational presentations, but as his work became more demanding, I often went alone or with a person living with AIDS. Often AIDS education became an avenue for pastoral care as well as an opportunity for a PWA to contribute to the educational outreach of the network. I often invited a PWA to tell his or her story either during training sessions for volunteers or when we conducted educational workshops in other settings. There certainly was overlap between pastoral care and spirituality, but the two functioned in different ways within the ministry of the network.

John, a PWA, often went with me to tell his story and respond to questions following an educational workshop in a congregation. I wrote the following letter in his memory for his memorial service.

Dear John,

How well I remember the day you walked into my office for the first time. That was almost two years ago. Although we had not met before, I did not feel like you were a complete stranger. Your former pastor had called me several months earlier to tell me about you. He cared deeply for you. You know all about that. You were thankful for his concern. But I have digressed.

You walked into my office that day and into my life. You entered tall and strong. I knew immediately that you were going to be in charge. No one that took you for granted or tried to tell you how to live your life would be allowed in close. That was fine with me. I like people who know what they want and can say so. By the time that first conversation ended, I had decided that if it was all right with you, I wanted to be your pastoral friend and companion on this dreadful, awesome journey we were undertaking. I respect those who can look at their circumstances and decide to participate actively in what will happen along the way rather than to sit by passively.

One thing that struck me that day was how determined you were to make your life count for something special during whatever time you had left. You said you wanted to help with the work of APCN. I didn't make it easy for you, John. I told you if you wanted to speak for APCN you had to go through our volunteer training and you would have to come listen to several presentations I made for the network. I wanted you to know what you were getting into. You took the challenge on both counts. Later you helped in the educational outreach of APCN. On a number of occasions, we worked as a team presenting important aspects of APCN's education and pastoral care. You were articulate and had a style that drew your listeners into your experience in helpful ways. I could tell how important it was to you to share your life with others as well as how much it meant to them. It brought meaning into your pain. I thank you for all you gave me in giving to others.

I remember lunch with you and your life partner Pete. Everything was beautiful and just right. One day you came to my office bringing me an early touch of spring with a lovely bouquet of tulips. You were interested in my life too, not only in what was happening to you. I became pastor and friend. I valued your ability to show me the many sides of yourself. You could be angry, complaining, demanding, fearful, tender, warm, affectionate, searching, vulnerable, strong, hopeful, and loving. John, I loved your honesty, all you were and all you shared with me. I have been blessed in this journey with you.

I remember your enthusiastic support for the AIDS WALK—a major fund-raiser for the AIDS agencies in Chicago—a year ago. You and your family worked so hard recruiting walkers and contributing to APCN in other ways. The relationship with APCN became a two-way ministry—we gave to you and you gave to us. Thank you John; may you rest in peace in God's presence. At its best, pastoral support of someone with

AIDS was as much a gift to the volunteer as to the person living with AIDS.

Brian

Brian was a young man I met through my volunteer work at Howard Brown Clinic and a person I continued to relate to while working with APCN.

I first met Brian when he was in his early twenties as he mourned the death of his mother. He was concerned about his reaction to her death. Although he missed her terribly, he could feel or express little emotion. He was numb. When he told me the number of his friends who had died, his reaction to his mother's death became understandable. Multiple losses within a short time can easily cause emotional overload and leave a person numb.

Brian and I had been meeting weekly for several months when I noticed one evening that he was unusually pale, chilling, and had a hacking cough. I suspected these were early symptoms of HIV infection. The following week I sat at his bedside as he waited to go to surgery for a bronchoscopy, which confirmed the diagnosis.

I visited him regularly over the next two years. In one of our visits he said he was considering suicide as a way out. As we explored the basis for his thoughts and interest, he admitted that he was afraid of dying alone. So many of his close friends were already gone, he wasn't sure anyone would be present with him at the time of death. Then and there I promised that if at all possible I would be with him when his time came.

Young as he was and with a history of "living in the fast lane," he became politically active. He was determined to do whatever he could to help provide better care for others with AIDS. It was a matter of great pride to him that he became an advocate for disability insurance, housing assistance, and Medicaid for PWAs. He was also successful in securing public assistance for the poor unable to afford AZT, a new drug with promise to slow down the progression of HIV infections. Brian, like many others, had found a purpose in life, a way to make a contribution to others, thus making his life count.

He participated several times with APCN volunteer training sessions, telling his story of living with AIDS. He went with me to our seminary in Elkhart, Indiana, after I was invited to speak about AIDS to a class of seminarians. He shared his story and responded to their questions during the discussion. It was amazing to notice the growth and maturity in his presentations as he lived with AIDS. I promised him if I ever wrote a book about my work, his story would be included.

Brian asked several times that I be called when he was hospitalized and thought his death was close. Each time I went to be with him. When a third call came at 1:30 a.m., the nurse assured me it was no false alarm. As quickly as I could, I got up and dressed for the forty-five-minute drive from my home to the hospital. Brian was still conscious when I arrived but weak and miserable, ready to let go. I stayed at the bedside frequently emptying his emesis basin at the sink in his room. I took the basin to the sink one moment, turned back toward him the next, and he was gone. The veil between life and death seemed as delicate as gossamer. I waited in the hospital until a reasonable hour of the morning before going to the home of Brian's father to notify him that Brian had died. Brian's mother had died several years earlier.

It was gratifying to see that as the work of APCN and the need for volunteers became known, many people wanted to volunteer: clergy, laypeople, and members of religious orders. The network provided the structure, opportunity, training, and guidance and support for the volunteers.

A committee helped screen and train volunteers. "Goodwill is not enough" soon became shorthand to indicate that not everyone who applied was accepted as a volunteer. We wanted to be sure each person had the capacity to listen and be present to the PWA without judgment. We also wanted the volunteer to be aware of and comfortable with his or her spiritual journey, able to listen and converse with a client who wanted to explore and nurture his or her own spirituality. At the same time we wanted to extend the same sensitivity toward potential volunteers that we expected of them. When a person's gifts and skills did not fit the needs of APCN, I suggested an alternate AIDS agency where their skills could be used.

One way we determined which volunteers had the aptitude and skills we wanted was to have each person share his or her spiritual journey within a small group of other applicants and a member of the APCN team. We were alert to ways the prospective volunteers related to each other and to members of the leadership team during the training sessions. Did they listen to each other and respond appropriately, did they seem defensive, self-serving, or self-denigrating? Were they sensitive to the feelings of others? During my five years with the organization, we saw few potential volunteers that I referred to other agencies.

It was my responsibility to match a volunteer with a PWA. I also chose to provide direct care for at least two people with AIDS at all times since I wanted to stay abreast of the kinds of situations our volunteers faced.

The following story is one example of the changes that could occur in a client during the pastoral-care relationship.

Larry

Larry was a small man in his mid-thirties when I first met him. He appeared fragile, full of sorrow and heartbreak because of his lover's recent death. The two had been partners for months instead of years, but Larry spoke of feeling closer to him than he had felt to anyone in his life. He was especially wounded because his lover's family took him back into the family in another city to care for him during the final weeks of his life. Larry had no way of bringing satisfying closure to the relationship.

He came to me weekly and for many months for bereavement counseling. He was one of the most negative people I have met. He complained that his roommate was selfish, his own work dull, his coworkers critical, his friends self-centered. He saw something wrong in every person he met and in every aspect of his life.

Eventually he became severely depressed and suicidal. Each week I asked him to promise that if he got to the place that he felt unable to go on, he would call me before harming himself. Each week he promised, then one evening he called. We talked at length. I was no longer comfortable taking full responsibility for someone so seriously depressed and sought the counsel of a therapist. She gave me the name of a psychiatrist, and I referred him for evaluation and possible medication.

Later Larry took another lover and moved to a distant city. When they came to Chicago for a visit, he and his lover stopped in to see me. The relationship was short-lived, and he returned to the Chicago area. In the meantime he had been diagnosed HIV positive and the infection soon became full-blown AIDS.

When he contacted me again, I asked if he was open to having a pastoral volunteer relate to him on a regular basis. He agreed, though he did not consider himself religious. I assigned a young Roman Catholic seminary student. They worked well together, and I did not see Larry for some time. But I always knew he would get in touch when he was ready.

When the time came for his pastoral companion to take his final vows for the priesthood, he invited Larry to the service. Later, as Larry described seeing his friend lying prostrate, with his face to the floor in an act of complete submission and availability to God, I heard the awe in his voice as he said, "I have never seen anything like that."

Larry had periods of illness interspersed with times when he was able to work, but he knew the end was somewhere just around the corner. He took the initiative to reconcile with his mother, from whom he had been estranged for a long time.

A rapidly growing tumor had invaded his chest, and his doctor suggested daily radiation treatments to keep him more comfortable. My office was located next door to the hospital where he received the treatments. Often he took the elevator up to the fifth floor to see if I was occupied with someone else. If my door was open he came in to chat for a few minutes, then went on his way.

One day I received a call that Larry had been admitted to the hospital next door. I went to see him. As we chatted I asked, "Larry, what do you see for yourself down the road?"

"Well," he said matter-of-factly, "I know I'm going to die and I'm going to see God. I have no regrets. I have the most wonderful friends anyone could have."

He appeared to be at peace, not anxious or fearful or fretful. The change was dramatic when compared to the person I remembered meeting several years earlier. Shortly after that conversation, Larry was discharged to go home to the apartment of a friend who was caring for him. I called his friend to set a time for me to visit. Much to my surprise, Larry was up walking around when I arrived. We sat at the kitchen table, where he asked if I would help with his memorial service. I promised to help if I was in town, but Larry crossed that delicate boundary between life and death a short time later, while I was away on vacation. I was sad to be unable to fulfill his last request.

Larry's roommate came to my office after I returned from vacation. He told me Larry had been unresponsive most the morning on the day of my last visit and had slipped back into unresponsiveness almost immediately after I left. We had been gifted with a little window in which to say our good-bye.

When I remember his bereavement and vulnerability, his depression and estrangement from his family, and finally his growth into peacefulness, I'm so grateful to have had a small part in his journey. I am especially thankful for APCN and the volunteer who gave Larry many hours of time and care. Writing his story so many years later still touches my heart.

♣

Our emphasis on spirituality was guided by several other professionals working with me to plan specific events to support individuals and the larger community as they grieved and searched for healing amid the terrible loss and suffering. Our APCN committee, in cooperation with another AIDS service provider, planned the annual interfaith memorial liturgy to be celebrated on the evening of Memorial Day. The interfaith service was one place where people bereft of their loved ones could gather as a community to express their faith through music, prayers, Scripture, other appropriate readings, and storytelling.

Equally important was their opportunity to express their grief in a tangible way. Huge banners hanging at the front of the sanctuary were taken down so that bereaved people could come forward and inscribe onto the banners the names of loved ones who had died. This was followed with a time of prayer, naming loved ones who were ill or had died. The service validated the relationships and commemorated the lives of loved ones. As the AIDS epidemic in the Chicago area grew, attendance at the liturgies grew as well until 600-800 people participated. After the service, participants went on a candlelight walk through the area of the city where the celebration was held.

People grieving the death of a loved one because of AIDS carried an exceptionally heavy burden during the crisis years. Shame and stigma silenced people whose loved ones had died. I sat in the church sanctuary one Sunday morning after leading an adult Christian education workshop on AIDS in a sophisticated mainline congregation in a Chicago suburb. As we waited for worship to begin, a young woman leaned close and whispered that her brother had died of AIDS two years earlier. "I have never told anyone about his death, not even my pastor." How tragic! What a burden to carry alone for two long years!

During a workshop for pastors and church leaders in California, a man told the story of an uncle who had died of AIDS several years earlier. "Since the day of his burial my uncle's name has never been mentioned in the family." I often pondered how or if people could possibly heal as long as they carried their grief in silence.

By the late 1980s the crisis had become so great that the annual memorial service, important as it was, could not the meet the needs of the large numbers of grieving people. Gay relationships were not valued or validated in the first place, so how could they grieve the deaths of their beloved partners? Where could they safely share their loss and pain? Support was almost nonexistent within communities of faith or in society in general. The most prevalent attitude was, "They are getting what they deserve." Many men were afraid to ask for time off work when a life partner died for fear of losing their jobs if the boss discovered they were gay. Occasionally a gay man returned from work to find his belongings on the sidewalk in front of the place where he had been living. The landlord or lady had discovered the person was gay. It was a very tough time.

Most of the dying were young, or in the prime of life. One death followed another in quick succession, leaving little time for friends, family, lovers, or life partners to heal before another friend died. A young man described his life and friendships as a jigsaw puzzle in which one piece after another had been popping out until little of the original design was left. Multiple losses in quick succession often result in a logjam of grief that blocks the emotions until the person becomes numb and lifeless. Depression is common.

As the crisis escalated the staff at APCN made a decision to offer grief support groups. My preference was to have eight to ten people in a group for six consecutive weeks. I interviewed every person before accepting them into a group. There was no problem finding the people. They came from all over Chicago and the surrounding suburbs. I found facilitating those support groups to be some of the most satisfying work I did. Significant healing often took place within the six weeks. Grieving was not completed within that period, but participants had been introduced to various tools that could help them continue their grief work. In addition group members often connected with each other and remained in contact after the formal group ended.

Originally the groups were open to gay men only, but later I asked myself where mothers, sisters, or women friends were to find support in their grieving. I invited several women into one of the groups, at first as an experiment. I was surprised to see the healing that took place when a mother was able to relate to a gay man in the group in ways she had never been able to relate to her own son. On other occasions the situation was reversed: a young man found healing because of a special bond he formed with a mother in the group. For a variety of reasons, it was sometimes more appropriate to work individually with a person rather than in the group. I was prepared to offer individual grief support when it seemed the best option. Our support groups certainly did not meet the needs of everyone but became an important source of healing for many.

Another task of the spirituality committee was to provide opportunities for individual clients to explore their own spirituality. Or to say it another way, to search for meaning within themselves or within a tradition they had left behind. Often they could integrate aspects of their early faith traditions in new ways that provided spiritual support as they lived day by day with the reality of a terminal illness.

The last three years I was with APCN the spirituality committee planned a weekend retreat at Lake Geneva, Wisconsin, for people who were HIV positive. A member of the spirituality committee served as a facilitator for some of the activities during the retreat. She led a guided meditation on Saturday morning inviting participants to focus on how they felt when they first learned they were HIV positive. She invited them to think about expressing their first reaction in terms of color, texture, symbols, and images that portrayed their feelings.

After the guided meditation, the participants helped themselves to paper and colorful pens and found a quiet place to translate their feelings into drawings. Some of the drawings were complex, others very simple. When everyone had completed their work, all the drawings were laid out for others to see; but no one was free to venture any kind of interpretation or judgment of another's work. Instead each person was invited to interpret what his or her drawing represented.

One drawing I found particularly poignant was simple, a large teardrop. That was all. As I recall, it represented the whole of the person's life after HIV. Life enclosed within a single teardrop. Another young man had drawn a vase with four flowers. One of the flowers drooped over the side of the vase, wilted. When asked what the drawing represented, he said the three beautiful flowers were his three sisters and the fourth "sickly" bloom was his own self.

The image of the person in the bed had been done in black and white, except for a swirl of vivid colors in the lower right-hand corner. The person who described the drawing avoided using any God language in his interpretation. He said there are pinholes in the universe that each of us must pass through, and on the other side is beauty. These exercises were powerful and moving for staff and participants alike.

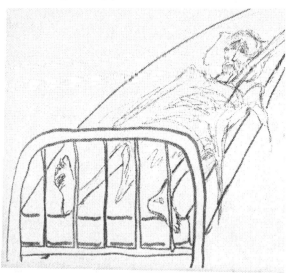

26

2004

The Legacy I Received

My work as a volunteer with Howard Brown Memorial Clinic and my five years with APCN allowed me to draw close to many people. The network provided the structure through which my urgency to discover what it means to grow up gay or lesbian in our culture and within the American religious scene was realized. I met hundreds of gay men and listened to countless stories of their life experiences. Many were heartrending stories of men who had once been capable seminarians, priests, pastors, youth group leaders, teachers, musicians, or lay members active in the church and the community. Many were afraid of "coming out of the closet," fearing harassment, humiliation, rejection, or loss of a job or housing, or sometimes physical injury. Others were estranged from the church because another person had revealed their secret and their worst fears had become stark reality. Usually such people were quickly dismissed from their jobs without recourse or due process.

Seminary students came for conversation, sometimes weeping their hearts out because they knew their chances of ever being ordained were almost nonexistent even if they promised to be celibate. Yet, like any of us, they craved human love and companionship. They longed to build solid relationships within the context of the church, with the support of a community of faith. Many had wonderful gifts for ministry. The church has been the loser. Frequently I pondered how it was possible that so many young people of unique and mysterious sexual identity (in the sense that all sexual identity is unique and mysterious) continued to yearn to be part of the church despite all the wounds the church has inflicted.

A profound shift occurred as I met so many gifted people and observed their commitment to each other through a most difficult time. I visited and spoke in churches whose primary membership was gay and lesbian and attended fellowship groups that met regularly for worship and mutual support.

Initially all our clients with APCN were gay men; however, within a few years that had changed. I met numerous women, a few who were married and had contracted AIDS because the husband had been using drugs and transmitted the virus to his wife. Sometimes a husband who considered himself heterosexual contracted the virus through occasional intimate contacts with gay men. Then there were the husbands, like mine, who were gay or bisexual and lived secret lives and became infected through numerous sexual encounters.

Children were not exempt from the suffering caused by HIV infection. Their lives were cut short because the insidious virus had been transmitted from mother to child. One young woman with a lengthy history of substance abuse entered a treatment facility when she discovered she was pregnant. She completed the program successfully and accepted motherhood eagerly. To her dismay her child had been infected with HIV, which meant the mother was HIV positive. Her child died before reaching age three. The mother was grief-stricken. She and her live-in companion, also in recovery, decided to care for infants with AIDS whose mothers were unable to care for them.

I had the opportunity to speak to thousands of people in churches, synagogues, universities, seminaries, high schools, and pastors' groups, offering workshops on the basics of HIV infection. Particularly within seminaries, pastors' groups, and congregations, I included an emphasis on pastoral care. In many if not most of those settings there were at least a few people who expressed the attitude that people with AIDS in the gay community were "guilty" and the rest were "innocent."

The educational work during those five years enlarged my vision and left an indelible imprint. Gradually, I learned that no matter the denomination or faith tradition, there were usually a few people in the crowd who thought the gay community was getting what it deserved in being decimated by AIDS. To hear those sentiments expressed again and again helped me realize just how ingrained and pervasive those attitudes are in the church. I saw that in regard to homosexuality and HIV, the church reflects the attitudes prevalent in society more accurately and to a greater extent than the attitude and response of Jesus to the outcasts of his day. I was and still am often saddened and incensed by the lack of compassion in the church.

My work with APCN, though often physically and emotionally draining, was at the same time satisfying. Throughout the five years board members were perceptive and responsive to the needs of the staff. I never sensed that they expected more of any staff member than was reasonable. I was trusted and always respected as a fellow professional. Board members expressed appreciation readily and frequently. I learned a great deal about the importance of fairness, honesty, respect, and appreciation in creating a positive atmosphere in the workplace. Most of that learning was readily applicable in the congregational settings where I have worked after leaving APCN.

I come from a faith tradition that prides itself on putting faith into action. Service is a primary watchword among us. That we are to serve others is so ingrained that we rarely see ourselves as needy. Until recently we rarely put ourselves into a position of learning with and receiving from other folk. I applaud and value my tradition's emphasis on service; however, my exposure to and work within the community so ravaged by AIDS from 1985 until 1991 taught me that Mennonites do not have a corner on service.

There was a great host of volunteers—hundreds of them—in the gay community who spent thousands of hours shopping, cooking, cleaning, changing bed linens, shaving, cutting hair, creating parties, seeing to every detail of the needs of their "brothers" who were suffering the horrible devastation of AIDS. It was not unusual for a man to take a leave of absence from his work to care for his dying partner. They exhibited the kind of commitment that when present among heterosexual people we admire as outstanding.

I often thought about the ministry of Jesus as he touched physically and emotionally those who were forced to live on the margins of society by the respectable people of his day. Jesus did not hesitate to touch the ritually unclean or to bless children, and to reach out to those needing healing. Jesus' circle of love was large enough to include them all. I feel certain that if Jesus had been in Chicago in person during the AIDS crisis, or today for that matter, he would be tending the sick, comforting the grieving, listening to the heartbroken, and sitting with the dying.

I remember a story about the kingdom that Jesus told as recorded in Matthew 25:31, 34-40:

> When the Son of man comes in his glory, and all the angels with him, then he will sit on the throne of his glory. . . . Then the king will say to those at his right hand, "Come, you that are blessed by my Father, inherit the kingdom prepared for you from the foundation of the world; for I was hungry and you gave me food, I was thirsty and you gave me something to drink, I was a stranger and you welcomed me, I was naked and you gave me clothing, I was sick and you took care of me, I was in prison and you visited me." Then the righteous will answer him, "Lord, when was it that we saw you

hungry and gave you food, or thirsty and gave you something to drink? And when was it that we saw you a stranger and welcomed you, or naked and gave you clothing? And when was it that we saw you sick or in prison and visited you?" And the king will answer them, "Truly I tell you, just as you did it to one of the least of these who are members [brothers and sisters] of my family, you did it to me."

Our little congregation in Oak Park was a source of encouragement and strength during those years. After a year studying many issues related to same-sex orientation, we became a congregation that welcomed gay and lesbian folk into membership. I found it particularly gratifying that our pastor and several laypeople invested a great deal of time and effort to help establish an organization in Oak Park to provide a variety of AIDS services. I would have been hard-pressed to find a more supportive congregation anywhere.

Through these rich and varied experiences with APCN, my supportive congregation, and the interior work of the Holy Spirit, I was being healed of my severe grief. And I certainly gained a deeper understanding of Ray and his life. Moreover, I can say with thanksgiving that writing this book has been instrumental in another level of healing my inner turmoil.

I have given you a glimpse into my work with those affected by HIV/AIDS. The AIDS scene I have described has changed dramatically in this country. I have friends who have been HIV positive for more than fifteen years and are doing well. They are leading full, productive lives because of medications that control the virus.

Unfortunately the same is not true in the poverty-stricken countries around the world where effective drugs are not available.

The statistics projected by the World Health Organization about fifteen years ago are a reality in those countries today. The earlier warnings fell on politically deaf ears in our country, and the same was true for most of the American church, including my own denomination. Recently our relief and development agency has been soliciting funds for the AIDS crisis in Africa. I'm grateful for that, but it is coming late in the season of the epidemic. There is an ache in my chest and I feel almost wordless from the report of 6,000 AIDS-related deaths in Africa every day. The horror is too great to contemplate—one million orphans in Uganda alone. Fields are empty of crops and become burial grounds because there is no one to plant and harvest crops.

I hurt anew when I remember the lack of support available for AIDS in this country during the 1980s. It seems easier to give money when the needs are far removed from our lives than it is to move beyond the safe boundaries that prevent us from reaching out here at home. Does Jesus weep over the church in our country today as he wept over Jerusalem?

My life was changed profoundly by Ray's illness and death and by my work during the years that followed. I hope I have become more understanding and compassionate, nonjudgmental, more ready to listen with the heart and more open to people whose lives touch mine.

I left the Chicago area and AIDS ministry in October 1991 to join the pastoral staff of First Mennonite Church in Denver, Colorado. It was my great joy to minister there for almost five years and since then to have served three additional Mennonite congregations as interim pastor. In each place I have listened to the pain of parents as they wrestled with the "coming out" of a gay son or daughter. It has also been my privilege to relate to young men and women who are gay or lesbian. Wives trying to cope with the discovery of a husband who is gay have also contacted me to listen and offer support. The painful and complex issues related to same-sex orientation and mixed-orientation marriage will continue to affect many, many people.

It is important to me to be part of a congregation that is inclusive, though that is not always an easy place to find. I am troubled and saddened by the increasingly strident voices in the church at large around issues of inclusion or exclusion. The last few years have been extremely painful because I have loved the church for many years and still do. I have found life-giving faith, purpose, and ministry in the church yet find it difficult not to be disillusioned by the intensity of the conflict today in my denomination. May God have mercy and lead us to love God with heart, soul, mind, and strength and our brothers and sisters as we love ourselves.

27

2004

Gratitude and Blessing

Reviewing the details of my life to make this story accessible to others has been satisfying, heartwarming, and at times heart-wrenching. Through the writing I have relived my life with Ray, including our seven-week journey from his diagnosis until his death. This process has effected a new depth of integration. All that has happened will continue to become more fully integrated into the person I will become in the future.

I see more clearly the complex interweaving of the wounds and the strengths we brought to our marriage—Ray's awareness of his sexual orientation, my naivete and limited sense of self. Ray's intelligence and his commitment to achieving his goals became positive gifts, yet sometimes hindered wholesome family life. The basic differences in our personalities and our histories meant we perceived the world and our stance in the larger world differently. We could not share perceptions and experiences of God easily. Both of us lacked the communication skills needed to negotiate our differences in helpful ways. Together we created our relationship with the tools at hand in the best way we could. All the raw materials were interwoven to create the life we lived. It is neither desirable nor possible to claim this or that was his fault or my fault. Both of us contributed to making our life together what it became. I am thankful for having shared my life with Ray. I am grateful for the possibility that exists to transform tragedy and defeat into new life, wholeness, peace, love, and contentment.

In many ways Ray and I were ill prepared to face our struggles; in another way we had what was most important, strong foundations of faith. I am amazed that growing up in our Amish home prepared me in quite surprising ways to relate to gay and lesbian folk. I knew firsthand what it was like to live on the margins of mainstream society. Never fitting in was familiar to me. In the 1930s and 1940s when I was growing up, Amish folk were not as well known or as respected in the larger society as they are today. Instead of living with a fearful secret, I always felt overexposed because there was no way to hide my unadorned, plain clothing. I worked long and hard to overcome the German accent I had when learning to speak English in elementary school. My being different was external but left me always aware that I did not really belong.

Another plus of growing up in our family was the complete openness with which my parents welcomed anyone into our home and to our table. Their welcoming spirit somehow found its way into my heart. I did not find it difficult to feel compassion for those affected by AIDS or to relate to people who were different from me in background and culture. It is possible that some folk who read this book may be offended by the parallel I have drawn between the hospitality of my parents and my response to people with AIDS and others in the gay and lesbian community. Nevertheless, it is clear to me that the openness of my parents set a dynamic precedent that affected my choices many years later.

Through God's abundant grace my life pilgrimage has crossed the paths of many caring people. It is also grace that at times I took the initiative to seek the guidance of such people. My blessed life has been a cooperative enterprise between God and my response to God's touch of grace and love. Living within communities of grace-filled, loving, supportive people has given me hope and strength and has relieved my sense of aloneness and isolation.

I am amazed at the way the disparate threads of my life have been woven together to create a tapestry from the muted tones of sadness, regret, anger, loss, and yearning intermingled with the bright colors of resurrection, love, joy, peace, hope, forgiveness, contentment, and trust. I now see that, even in the most difficult times, God was always present. It was my limited knowledge and understanding of the Infinite One and my pain that often kept me too self-absorbed to be aware of God's presence day by day.

At this point it seems that my whole life had been a preparation for Ray's illness that led to his death and my ministry that has followed. I now claim as gift all that my life has been and all it is becoming each day. I have no illusions about the future being without challenges and perhaps even great suffering, yet I hope to embrace with grace and courage whatever the future holds.

A Prayer

Creator God, you have touched my life with grace from my earliest beginnings. The parents who gave me birth laid a strong foundation of faith, a faith that through the years has been tested, molded, and shaped by the changes and challenges, the possibilities and predicaments, the trials and sufferings common to daily living. It was pure grace that opened my heart to the beauty and mystery of life in Jesus Christ. God, you have shown me glimpses of grace through my relationships with siblings, teachers, pastors, friends, communities of faith, and especially through our children.

You have blessed me beyond measure, and I give you thanks.

Redeeming God, it was your gift of grace that brought Ray

and me together in order for each of us to do the inner work necessary to become the persons you created us to become. You have given me glimpses of your love and grace shining through all our incompleteness, imperfections, and weaknesses. Ultimately your grace broke through the protective barriers of fear that had separated us and brought us into the light of honesty, truth, freedom, and love.

You have blessed me beyond measure, and I give you thanks.

Empowering God, I praise you for all those who planted seeds in my heart, seeds that took root and grew slowly, silently until they yielded a harvest of love. It was your spirit that beamed your grace into my life through Ray's friends and the countless people who contributed to my life during the years of my search to understand those who had been "strangers" to me. With a touch of grace you empowered and entrusted me with a ministry of compassion.

You have blessed me beyond measure, and I give you thanks.

Whispering God, it was your whispers of grace and the audible voices of your people that led me into ministry in congregations of the Mennonite Church. In those communities of faith you have shown yourself loving and able to heal human misery, pain, and discouragement.

You have blessed me beyond measure, and I give you thanks.

Sustaining God, it is surely your grace that has kept me through all the years of my life. You have sustained me as I have written this story, a story written for the sake of Ray and me, and our children. Most of all, O God, I have written the story for your sake because my story has become part of the Story you have given to the world as a gift of pure love and grace.

I pray that the Story will live in my children and the children of the future generations of our family. It is not the details of my particular story that will go on and on but the miracle of the God-and-human Story that will continue throughout all time.

May it be so.

Notes

1. This chapter on Ray's early years is abbreviated to protect siblings still living.

2. Henri J. M. Nouwen, *Bread for the Journey: A Daybook of Wisdom and Faith* (San Francisco: HarperSanFrancisco, 1997), reading for June 20.

3. Ed was estranged from the church for many years. He wrote his psalmlike prayer/poem as death from AIDS was drawing near. It was written in his diary near Christmas 1986. Used by permission of his mother, Nancy Byrnes Riley.

The Author

From Ann Showalter's early teens into marriage and mother-hood, a dynamic faith characterized her life. She cared for their family of four children and worked part-time while the children were in school. She was also active in the community, serving a three-year term on the local school board and the board for special education.

Active participation in the local church was always important in Ann's life. Singing in church choir, teaching, serving on the church council and in other leadership roles, became the visible signs others read as gifts pointing toward seminary and ordained ministry. After their children left home, Ann went to seminary, graduating with a Masters of Divinity in 1982 and was ordained to the ministry in 1984.

Her birth into an Old Order Amish family on a farm near Kokomo, Indiana, seemed light years away from the Chicago hospital the afternoon her husband revealed his hidden life as a gay man. His death from AIDS seven weeks later was the impetus for Ann's ministry with others affected by the AIDS crisis. It was a ministry that led her to question the traditional views and attitudes of the church and society toward same-sex orientation.

Currently Ann is retired and lives in Newton, Kansas where she worships with the New Creation Fellowship Church. She offers individual spiritual direction and occasionally leads workshops at Heartland Center for Spirituality in Great Bend, Kansas

Printed in the United States
45780LVS00007B/106-120